Inner-City Nephrology

Onyekachi Ifudu (ed)

ISBN: 1-4140-3651-5 (e-book)
ISBN: 1-4140-3652-3 (Paperback)

This book is printed on acid free paper.

Edited by
Onyekachi Ifudu, M.D., M.Sc
Associate Professor of Medicine
Director, Inpatient Dialysis Services
SUNY Downstate Medical Center, Brooklyn, New York

1st Books - rev. 02/24/04

Dedication

To my parents, for their unconditional love.

Table of Contents

List of Main Authors

Onyekachi Ifudu, M.D., M.Sc *Editor*
Associate Professor of Medicine
Director, Inpatient Dialysis Services
SUNY Downstate Medical Center
Are Turf Battles and Managed Care To Blame For Late Referral of ESRD Patients?

Gerald Appel, M.D.
Professor of Medicine
Director of Clinical Nephrology
Nephrology Division
Columbia University College of Physicians & Surgeons
622 West 168th Street
Attn: Transplant Dialysis Office, Room 4128
New York, NY 10032
Hyperlipidemia in Kidney Disease: Effects on Disease Progression and Mortality

Clive O. Callender, M.D., F.A.C.S.
LaSalle D. Leffall Jr., Professor of Surgery
Chairman, Department of Surgery
Director, Transplant Center
Howard University Hospital
2041 Georgia Ave. N.W.
Washington, DC 20060
Strategies To Maximize Organ Donation In The Inner-City

Neil R. Powe, MD, MPH, MBA
Director, Welch Center for Prevention, Epidemiology and Clinical Research
Professor of Medicine, Epidemiology and Health Policy & Management
The Johns Hopkins Medical Institutions

2024 E. Monument Street, Suite 2-600
Baltimore, MD 21205-2223
Do For-Profit Dialysis Companies Care More About Profits Than Patients?

Robert Provenzano, M.D.
Chief, Division of Nephrology
Associate Clinical Professor of Medicine
Department of Internal Medicine
St John Hospital and Medical Center
Detroit, Michigan 48236
Optimizing Anemia Management in Chronic Kidney Disease

Iram Anees, M.D.
Senior Transplant Fellow
Renal Disease Division
SUNY Downstate Medical Center, Brooklyn, New York
Gynecologic and Reproductive Concerns In ESRD

Clinton Brown, M.D.
Assistant Professor of Medicine
Director, Ambulatory Dialysis Center
& Hyperlipidemia Clinic
Gender and Race Discrimination in US Uremia Therapy: What is The Truth?

Barbara Delano, M.D., M.P.H.
Professor of Medicnine
Director, Home Hemodialysis & CAPD
SUNY Downstate Medical Center, Brooklyn, New York
CAPD versus Hemodialysis: Which For The Urban Poor?

Eli A. Friedman, M.D., M.A.C.P
Distinguished Teaching Professor of Medicine
Chief, Renal Disease Division
SUNY Downstate Medical Center, Brooklyn, New York

Diabetes and Hypertension: An Inner-City Catastrophe

Anthony Joseph, M.D.
Assistant Professor of Medicine
Director, Ambulatory Nephrology Service
Renal Disease Division
SUNY Downstate Medical Center, Brooklyn, New York
Preventing Infections in ESRD – Are We Doing Enough?

Joan D. Mayers, R.N., C.N.N.
Assistant Director of Nursing
SUNY Downstate Medical Center, Brooklyn, New York
Is Dietary Counseling Effective In A Multicultural Setting?

T.K.S. Rao, M.D., F.A.C.P.
Professor of Medicine
Director, Impatient Dialysis Services
Kings County Hospital, Brooklyn, New York
Has HAART Slowed The Epidemic of HIV Nephropathy In The Inner-City?

Moro O. Salifu, M.D., F.A.C.P.
Assistant Professor of Medicine
Renal Disease Division
SUNY Downstate Medical Center, Brooklyn, New York
Racial Differences in Transplant Outcomes – Biology vs Socioeconomic Factors?

Yalem Woredekal, M.D.
Assistant Professor of Medicine
Director, Outpatient Dialysis Services
Kings County Hospital, Brooklyn, New York
Emergency Room Care of ESRD Patients – What NonNephrologists Need To Know

Introduction
Eli A. Friedman

Once linkage between hyperglycemia and progression or renal disease in diabetes was clearly established in 1987 by the Diabetes Control and Complication Trial [1], routine medical care of diabetic patients carried the physician responsibility to strive fro euglycemia. Similarly, as powerful antihypertensive drugs were shown to retard progression of kidney disorders in diabetic [2] and nondiabetic patients [3], a mandate to normalize hypertensive blood pressures materialized. Correction of the anemia of renal insufficiency may prove to be an additional measure to retard inexorable forward march of some kidney disease [4].

Combining these measures into a comprehensive regimen defines the beginning of "renoprotection [5]." Unexpectedly and remarkably, thinking about end-stage renal disease (ESRD) transformed from devising strategies to cope with a burgeoning problem in health care delivery to constructing programs to increase public awareness of undiagnosed and untreated hypertension and type 2 diabetes. With something beneficial to advise at periodic visits during the course of renal deterioration, nephrologists have increasingly assumed an activist posture in treating pre-end stage kidney disease. At the start of the twenty-first century, ESRD is a disorder for which prevention is more important than the wonderful therapies of dialysis and kidney transplantation.

From 1989 through 1994, Downstate Medical Center's Renal Disease Division of the Department of Medicine conducted annual teaching days addressed to clarification of what was labeled "Inner-City Nephrology". The intent and focus of these exercises was to examine unique problems of incidence, prevalence, and management of kidney disorders in poor urbanites. Consequent to Downstate's location in the heart of America's largest black community, these conferences stressed the impact of hypertension, diabetes, AIDS, and drug abuse. Documenting the reality that blacks have approximately 3.5 times greater risk of renal failure than do whites, nephrologists and other members of kidney teams have learned that in dialysis units in Brooklyn, Queens, and the Bronx (subdivisions of New York City) are filled with a large majority of black patients.

After a lapse of seven years, Dr. Onyekachi Ifudu revived the Inner-City Nephrology Conferences with an eye to broad dissemination of the message that there are special attributes to the demographics of kidney disease as seen in those constrained to live and die in big cities in America. Blending together ongoing research initiatives with clinical imperatives derived from patient care, the present volume freshly defines the challenge and opportunity confronting those who practice kidney care inside of cities. Dr. Ifudu deserves thanks for making evident how far we have come and where we must yet travel along the road to eliminating the extra toll of being poor and suffering kidney disease in the inner city.

Eli A. Friedman, M.D.

References

1. The Diabetes Control and Complications Trial (DCCT). Design and methodologic considerations for the feasibility phase. The DCCT Research Group. Diabetes 1986;35:530-45.
2. Walser M.Angiotensin-receptor blockers, type 2 diabetes, and renoprotection. N Engl J Med 2002;346:705-7.
3. Taal MW, Brenner BM.Evolving strategies for renoprotection: n on-diabetic chronic renal disease.Cur Opin Nephrol Hypertens 2001;10:523-31.
4. Jungers P, Choukroun G, Oualim Z, Robino C, Nguyen AT, Man NK. Beneficial influence of recombinant human erythropoietin therapy on the rate of progression of chronic renal failure in predialysis patients. Nelphrol Dial Transplant 2001;16:307-12.
5. Hebert LA, Wilmer WA, Falkenhain ME, Ladson-Wofford SE, Nahman NS Jr, Rovin BH. Renoprotection: one or many therapies? Kidney Int 2001;59:1211-26.

Diabetes and Hypertension: An Inner-City Catastrophe
Eli A. Friedman, M.D.

Introduction

Legal and ethical concerns generated in the practice of nephrology often provoke strong partisan debate [1,2]. Inner city kidney patients present issues common to affluent exurbanites plus specific problems spawned by their poverty and – for some – a furtive undocumented existence. Critics of the caliber of medicine practiced in the inner city fuse resentment over indignities imposed by indigence with actualities sired by the difficulty of maintaining an illegal presence in an increasingly computerized country.

Money drives the quality of health care. The World Health Organization (WHO)[3] tabulated annual individual income in reporting countries noting the contrast between $23,240 in the USA and $180 in Tanzania $180 where there is no ESRD therapy. Similarly, a quarter-century ago, the European Dialysis and Transplant Association (EDTA) demonstrated a direct relationship between a country's per capita income and the number of patients enrolled in ESRD therapy [4]. The EDTA registry stated: "It is difficult for countries with a gross national product (GNP) lower than 2,700 US dollars to put many patients on treatment. Three-quarters of the world's population live where the per capita GNP is below 2,700 US dollars."

A gage of the quality of health care is afforded by a country's infant survival rate. For example, of every 5 women giving birth in Senegal, 4 receive no professional medical care, resulting in a first-year infant mortality of 68 per 1,000 compared with 5.2 per 1,000 in Sweden. An obvious inference from WHO studies is that for the foreseeable future, the world will be unable to afford uremia therapy [5]. Nations too poor to afford physicians, safe water and supervised pregnancies are preempted from establishing renal failure programs matching America's cost in excess of $65,000 per patient per year [6]. Developing nations including Cambodia, Chad, Ethiopia, and Tanzania cannot divert funds to uremia therapy until basic survival is assured. Like a third world developing nation, residents of the inner city live with muted aspirations and goals. The point of the foregoing is that in the inner city, especially for noncitizens fearing discovery of their illegal presence, any discussion of an ethical approach to treating kidney failure must begin with appreciation of the constraints imposed by being poor and/or undocumented.

Rationing Renal Services in the Inner City

Retrospective studies in the United Kingdom [7,8] illustrate how acceptance for ESRD treatment can be regulated both by governmental policies and economic pressures [9]. A more subtle means of rationing is through non-referral of uremic patients by generalists and nephrologists to dialysis facilities [10,11]. Within the inner city, Kjellstrand warned that: added to the need to overcome government and physician restriction to patient referral for dialysis uremic patients requiring treatment face "not-so-subtle economic pressure by managed care, government, administrators, and politicians, is already in force [12]. While state Medicaid programs proffer "emergency" dialysis for every uremic patient presenting to a hospital, continuing dialysis therapy may be limited and organ transplants unsupported in the absence of a "Green Card."

Inner city residents, even US citizens, who are minority group members – particularly blacks – face inferior outcome when given a kidney transplant. As remarked by Young and Gaston, blacks "remain significantly disadvantaged in both access and outcomes compared with whites [13]." The complex explanation for a substandard outcome may lie in lower availability of living kidney donors, a high rate of single parenthood plus a high rate of comorbid conditions in the parental donor pool. Furthermore, there is a restriction on kidney donation by single parent mothers because "she tends to have numerous other dependents [14]."

Resorting to a "blame the victim" assessment, relatively poor kidney graft and patient survival in poor black kidney transplant recipients in Mississippi has been ascribed to "noncompliance with transplant medications [15] (vide infra). Whether or not blacks and other minority group members are less compliant with immunosuppressive drugs has been studied [16], with blacks scored as generally less compliant than European whites [17]. Empowered

2

by Callender [18], a Minority Organ Tissue Transplant Education Program (MOTTEP) [19] focuses on broad community-based programs designed to promote organ donation by blacks as well as the acceptance of kidney transplantation as a modality for treatment of ESRD that may be superior to dialysis. Relatively lower ESRD treatment rates in the inner city, especially by kidney transplantation, are thus based both on socioeconomics and on cultural differences that may yield to educational outreach initiatives as provided by MOTTEP.

Stress in Uremia Therapy

As is true for all life sustaining medical regimens, stress is an inherent component of ESRD therapy. Unique to the management of kidney failure, however, is an unremitting requirements for sophisticated patient participation, whether by altering daily plans to permit scheduled hemodialyses, aseptic performance of peritoneal dialysis fluid exchanges or scrupulous adherence to the dietary and medication schedule that sustains a transplanted kidney.

Only in America, is therapy for ESRD a universal entitlement by law and in practice. Incidence treatment rates in other industrialized nations are less than one-half that in the United States. Assuming equivalent indigenous endemic kidney disease rates, either the US treats too many or other nations by treating too few, permit the death of potentially salvageable uremic patients. In fact, except or the wealthiest nations, the reality is that everyone manifesting kidney failure cannot be treated by dialysis or a kidney transplant because of economic constraints [20] and a shortage of cadaver organs. Throughout the world, supply versus demand makes rationing of therapy for ESRD unavoidable [21].

Schemes to allocate scarce medical resources include scoring points for age, diagnosis, economic and/or political status (citizenship). Privileges in a capitalistic society is unequal. Wealthy individuals have the option of purchasing a living-donor kidney though marketing is furtive and often hidden [22]. The kidney patient requires allies when coping with the quest for ESRD therapy. Patient organizations like the American Association of Kidney Patients attempt education and group support. To the extent possible under local circumstances, the patient's interests are best served when personal physicians decide their fate.

Factors that limit Uremia therapy within and outside the Inner City

This essay concentrates on unique problems arising from being poor and a minority group member with kidney failure in the inner city. Those forces that impinge on kidney patients irrespective of residence within or outside the inner city while noted briefly will not be dissected. Beneath this context, restricted distribution of uremia therapy, including donor kidneys, is equally applied to the inner city when the patient has advanced age, is mentally deficient, or has a futile prognosis is equivalent.

Glover and Moss struggle to reach the conclusion that: "Rationing according to social worth, ability to pay, or age is not ethically justifiable, but it is justified to ration according to medical benefit [23]." Such reasoning dances around admitting the infirmity imposed by advanced age in that the medical benefit derived from a kidney transplant is greater for a forty-year old than a ninety-year old, all other factors being equivalent? The literature on the subject is, at the least, conflicted as exemplified by Nilstun and Ohlsson who advise: "Health care rationing by age is inconsistent with the principles of equality and liberty. But in some situations such rationing has support from the principles of solidarity and efficiency. The compromise suggested is that, as a rule, rationing by age should not be permitted, except in situations with intrinsic scarcity (as is the case with transplantation) and in situations with temporary extrinsic scarcity (as was the case with dialysis for a period of time) [24]." Penetrating the meaning of this passage might occupy a class of Talmudic scholars for weeks.

Increasingly, the geriatric ESRD patient calls it quits. Pulitzer Prize-winning author "Tales of the South Pacific" James M. Michener, at age 90, after three years of hemodialysis, articulated one aged patient's perspective. "A person on dialysis undergoes very heavy and irritating treatment and in time it seems more than you can bear. There's always an easy out, just don't go to the hospital. Then after two weeks, you're dead. For the first time I could understand how a person could say "'the hell with it.'" Michener died, days after ordering his doctors in Austin, Texas to stop dialysis [25].

Uncomprehending permanently mentally disabled patients, in the author's view, should not be begun on ESRD therapy. At variance with this assertion are reports of satisfactory ESRD treatment in Down's syndrome by kidney transplantation [26]. Ethical questions provoked by managing uremia in the marginally intelligent or mainly unaware are difficult. Similarly, proposed ESRD therapy should not be applied when a patient's condition is futile, meaning less than a 1% probability of reversing "permanent" unconsciousness and/or dependence on intensive medical care [27].

Responding negatively to requested dialysis therapy in inner city patients with no hope of recovery is not ethically different from declining the request from affluent families wanting the health care team to "do something." As life slips away, families express hope that a hemodialysis machine may accomplish a magical reversal in the downward course of a loved one. Extreme caution is appropriate when sentencing an ESRD patient to death by non-treatment on the basis of a futile prognosis.

Surprise may reverse even carefully drawn projection of the patient's course. Pushing the vanguard of therapy beyond what is currently conventional, constantly redefines who may or may not gain rehabilitation by ESRD therapy. Open minded nephrologists willing to go beyond consensus constraints successfully extended long-term dialysis to blind diabetics [28], and formerly universally excluded HIV positive individuals [29]. Continuing redefinition of who ought to receive treatment for ESRD under which circumstances is certain.

Noncompliant Patients

Minimal evidence sustains the assertion that inner city ESRD patients are less likely to comply with medical regimens than are more affluent city dwellers? What is known, is that behavior patterns that stretch the implied contract between patient and health care team are more common in the inner city [30]. Examples of diseases with greater inner city prevalence include: hypertension [31], tuberculosis [32], type 2 diabetes [33], alcoholism [34,35], drug addition [36], AIDS [37,38], and violent crime [39,40]. It follows that inner city kidney patient are exposed to an environment that nurtures resistance to the orderly living pattern necessitated by repetitive dialyses or continuous immunosuppression.

Noncompliance in dialysis patients is defined as: skipping one or more dialyses in a month, shortening by 10 or more minutes one or more dialyses in a month, an interdialytic weight gain of more than 5.7% or dry weight, or a serum phosphate (PO_4) of greater than 7.5 mg/dl [41]. Noncompliance manifested by antisocial or combatative behavior that fractures the doctor-patient relationship as an expression of the patient's admixture of fear, fatigue, and anxiety [42].

Expression of noncompliance may vary widely as listed in Table III. Routinely, both dialysis and transplant patients regularly exhibit noncompliance with dietary and/or medication prescriptions. Illustrating this point is the study by Greenstein and Siegal noting that at least one in five surveyed recipients of solid organ allografts omitted one or more doses of immunosuppressive medications [43]. Inappropriate overaggressive resposes to noncompliance in ESRD patients fosters an atmosphere of antagonism and a struggle that may defeat the physician's primary obligation to beneficence. Reacting to belligerent, threatening, law-suit-minded patients, nephrologists feeling besieged may attempt to break the patient-physician bond discharging the patient by any legitimate means. Sermon assessed the major ethical issues that must be addressed when responding to beliegernece and other threatening behavior by a dialysis patient [44].

Lundin acting in the dual roles of physician and dialysis patient advocated better teaching and communication to reduce noncompliance by dialysis patients, most frequently expressed by non-adherence to diet, medications, or the dialysis schedule [45]. Ignoring dietary restrictions, despite adverse consequences, is indicative of an attempt by the patient to regain control of his person in a dependent situation [46]. Lundin advised: "When the dialysis staff rises to the challenge of making the treatment comfortable as well as efficiently fitting it into the patient's life outside the unit there should be fewer intratreatment complications and premature signoffs."

Posed in Table IV, are six questions, the answer to which will synthesize an assessment of the genesis and possible resolution of a kidney patient's defiance and challenge to the health care team. With a formulation constructed, a remedy may emerge. An excellent guide for evaluating and managing noncompliant and abusive ESRD patients is proffered by Alvin H. Moss at West Virginia University [47].

Questions Helpful in Analyzing Noncompliant Behavior (Table IV)

Is the genesis of kidney failure understood? The majority of inner city ESRD patients, lacking basic medical care at all times, present with advanced irreversible renal insufficiency, late in the course of their disease without psychological preparation for ESRD [48]. Without medical guidance, any purported linkage between harmful conduct (alcoholism, heroin injections) and renal disease may be remote. Explaining that kidney failure may be the result of either hepatitis C or narcotic drug toxicity may be sufficient to cause a disruptive patient to go along with a disputed treatment plan.

Has the renal strategy been made clear? Without an understanding of how dialysis works or why it must be performed, few ESRD patients are able to recite the most recent results for their serum albumin, hematocrit, or dialysis efficiency (urea reduction rate or KT/V), though these numbers govern their present and forecast their future. Exactly why the dose of erythropoietin is to be raised or the length of dialysis treatments increased can be an obscure mystery rather than a step in patient participation.

Does the patient have the necessary intellect and motor skills to comply with treatment? A blind diabetic stroke patient cannot perform peritoneal dialysis fluid exchanges. Individuals with severe mental deficiency cannot modify insulin doses according to plasma glucose levels. Complicated treatment plans cannot be initiated in the absence of support from family or a partner. **Can support figures assist in reasoning with the patient?** Soliciting the help of a spouse, parent, child, friend or clergy person can bridge the gap between renal team and noncompliant patient.

Is the patient psychotic? Reasoning with a psychotic patient may be fruitless. Schizophrenia, bipolar disorders, and some rare enzyme deficiencies [49], like brain tumors may alter personality and precipitate aggressive and/or antisocial behavior.

Might noncompliant behavior be a quest for secondary gain? To obtain lodging and food during a cold northern winter, homeless individuals may posture as antisocial in order. By resisting occupational therapy and other rehabilitation programs, a dialysis patient may secure monthly disability checks that amount to a greater sum than might be earned at a low paying job for the unskilled.

Resolving Patient-Staff Confrontations (Table V)

Nephrology team members unprepared for "incidents" may react with confusion and as a consequence of their fluster, inflame and accelerate rather than calm and ameliorate patient agitation. The ten items in Table V can be distilled down to a single admonition: "Carefully listen to the patient's complaints and wants." The teaching of Theodore Reich in his incisive text: "Listening With the Third Ear [50]," underscored the necessity to be receptive to more than the words being spoken by a suffering individual. Often, a listener's receptive posture and body language will prompt the patient to reveal what is really wrong. A patient believing the listener to be empathetic may reveal that repetitive lateness for dialysis treatments is due to the patient's wait for a school bus for a disabled child before departing for the dialysis facility. It then becomes easy to fix the problem by scheduling the patient for a later shift.

Another example is the interpretation of an insensitive remark by a staff member interpreted as racial bias inducing smouldering resentment that surfaces as hostility. Again, the fix is easy requiring only determination of who said what and talk it through. Employing the technique of "reflective listening' the therapist signals having "heard" what another has said. Should reasoning misfire, with the intensity of patient anger increasing, the sequence outlined in Table VI, focuses specifically on abusive dialysis patients concluding that for competent individuals who "behave in dangerous ways.......suspension of dialysis would, in our judgment, have been ethically defensible [51].

Orenlicher, counsel for the American Medical Association instructs:: "The obligation to treat non-compliant patients should not be an absolute one [52]." On the other hand, attempting balance, the AMA counsel then warns: "Patients should not have to pay for their non-compliance with their lives." Recalling the resolution proposed by King Solomon who counseled two mothers claiming the same baby that the patient must be cut in half, the discharge-don't discharge instruction can stultify corrective action. To preserve the function of a dialysis unit under assault by an abusive noncompliant dialysis patient, transfer to another facility makes sense, *providing that the patient's welfare is protected.*

Unwanted by and embarrassing to the responsible nephrologist are

TABLE I

Vital Statistics (Selected: World Health Organization 1999

	Per Capita Annual Income (US $)	Literacy (%)	Safe Water (%)	Infant Mortality/ 1000 births	Attended Delivery (%)	% of Budget for Health Care	Life Expectancy at Birth (Years)
Brazil	2770	82.5	92	54	84	5.8	66.2
Cambodia	222	35.2	12.9	117	29	?	49
China	380	73.2	82.8	21.5	45.3	3.1	70
Egypt	630	51	83.7	33.3	33.5	5	64.7
Germany	23030	99	100	6.9	?	13.5	75.7
India	330	52.1	44.1	79	44.1	2.9	61.1
Italy	20460	97.4	100	8	100	8.3	77.2
Japan	23730	100	95	4.8	100	5.1	78.5
Senegal	650	32	43.5	68	20	5.8	53.3
Sweden	27010	99	100	5.2	100	8.8	78.3
Tanzania	180	90	49	92	53	2.1	53
United Kingdom	17790	99	100	6.6	98	6	76.4

| USA | 23240 | 99 | 100 | 8 | | 99 | 12.7 | 75.9 |

TABLE II

Variables in Acceptance for the Outcome of ESRD Treatment

Variable	Developing Nation	US Inner City
Personal Poverty	XXXX	XX
Citizenship	XX	XXXX
Advanced Age	XXX	X
Political Connection	XXXX	-
Race	X	X
Gender	XXX	½ X
Extensive Disability [59]	XXXX	XX
Vegetative State [60]	XX	XX
Advanced Psychiatric Disorder [61,62]	XXXX	XX

X = Minor, XX = Substantial, XXX = Major, XXXX = Dominant

TABLE III

Noncompliance in Kidney Patients

1. Missing visits, payments
2. Non-adherence to diet
3. Non-adherence to medications
4. Late arrival for scheduled visit or treatment
5. Omitting dialyses, terminating hemodialyses early
6. Proscribed behavior in treatment unit (eating on dialysis)
7. Verbal threats/abuse to healthcare team or support staff
8. Filing unsubstantiated complaints to State Health Department
9. Initiating unsubstantiated "nuisance" lawsuits against healthcare team
10. Disruptive action in treatment unit or clinic
11. Physical assault on healthcare team

TABLE IV

Assessing Noncompliant Behavior

1.   Does the patient realize the genesis of his kidney failure?
1.   Does the patient grasp the intent of renal therapy?
1.   Does the patient have the necessary intellect and motor skills to comply with treatment?
1.   Can support figures assist in reasoning with the patient?
2.   Is the patient psychotic?
3.   Is there secondary gain by noncompliant behavior?

Table V

Discern and Eliminate Reasons for Patient Non-compliance

1. Remove "communication spoilers," such as criticizing, name-calling, moralizing, threatening, ordering and psychologic diagnosing.
2. Employ "reflective listening," to show that the patient has been "heard."
3. Deal directly with problem behaviors: small steps, involve the patient, build on patient's strengths, be clear on who is to do what when.
4. Devise new approaches to "old problems," such as lateness and complaints.,
5. Detail the consequences of aberrant behavior in terms that are comprehensible.
6. Prepare a behavior contract that specifies what is to be done by patient and renal team.
7. Prepare in advance to manage anger.
8. Anticipate for the staff a step-by-step coping with agitated and disruptive patients.
9. Establish and publicize a grievance procedure.
10. Appoint a patient representative.

Table VI

When Reasoning Fails and Dialysis Patient Abuse of Staff Continues

1. Inventory potential third party problem solvers (spouse, family, friend, clergy, others).
2. Carefully document incidents and staff responses in the patient's chart.
3. Involve the unit social worker and obtain psychiatric consultation if indicated.
4. Report the growing problem to the unit or hospital "risk management" service.
5. Advise the patient **in writing by certified mail** that a limit in toleration of the patient's action has been defined. Establish a date for compliance.
6. Should the abusive behavior continue beyond the time limit, notify the patient of termination of services **in writing by certified mail** permitting sufficient time for the patient to seek and obtain alternative dialysis care (at least 30 days). Include in the notification a list of proximal dialysis units and the directors' phone numbers.

TABLE VII

Assessing Ethical Issues in Kidney Patients

1. Has all relevant medical information been reviewed?
2. Is patient capable of making medical decisions?
3. If not, who is appropriate decision maker?
4. Were decisions made by a surrogate? Justification?
5. Have advance directives been signed?
6. Have key parties met to discuss case?
7. Are there legal constraints?

References

1. Friedman EA.Must (should) all ESRD patients be treated. in Ethics and the Kidney (editor Normal G. Levinsky) Oxford University Press, Oxford 2001 pp 85-109.

2. Friedman EA. (Editor) Legal and Ethical Issues in Treating Kidney Failure. Case Study Manual. 2000, Kluwer, Dordrecht, The Netherlands.

3. World Health Organization Statistical Information System. 1999 Data Tables for 1996. WHO website, Geneva Switzerland April 12, 1999.

4. Jacobs C, Broyer M, Brunner FP, Brynger H, Donckerwolcke RA, Kramer P, Selwood NH, Wing AJ, Blake PH 1981 Combined report on regular dialysis and transplantation in Europe, XI, 1981. Proc Eur Dial Transplant Assoc Eur Ren Assoc;18:4-58.

5. Friedman EA. 1995 Facing the reality: The world cannot afford uremia therapy at the start of the 21st century. Artificial Organs;19: 481-485.

6. Bruns FJ, Seddon P, Saul M, Zeidel ML 1998 The cost of caring for end-stage kidney disease patients: an analysis based on hospital financial transaction records. J Am Soc Nephrol;9:884-890.

7. Berlyne GM 1982 Over 50 and uremic equals death. The failure of the British National Health Service to provide adequate dialysis facilities. Nephron;31:189-190.

8. Mallick NP 1997 The costs of renal services in Britain. Nephrol Dial Transplant;12 Suppl 1:25-28. United States Renal Data System, USRDS 1999 Annual Data Report, The National Institutes

of Health, National Institute of Diabetes and Digestive and Kidney Diseases. Bethesda, MD, August 1999.

9. Schena FP. 1997 Report on the first meeting of the Chairmen of the National and International Registries. Kidney Internat;52:1422.

10. McKenzie JK, Moss AH, Feest TG, Stocking CB, Siegler M. 1998 Dialysis decision making in Canada, the United Kingdom, and the United States. Am J Kidney Dis;31(1):12-18.

11. Mendelssohn DC, Kua BT, Singer PA. 1995 Referral for dialysis in Ontario. Arch Intern Med;155:2473-2478.

12. Kjellstrand CM. 1996 High-technology medicine and the old: the dialysis example. J Intern Med 1996;239:195-210.

13. Young CJ, Gaston RS. African Americans and renal transplantation: disproportionate need, limited access, and impaired outcomes. Am J Med Sci 2002;323:94-9.

14. Hidalgo G, Tejani C, Clayton R, Clements P, Distant D, Vyas S, Baqi N, Singh A.Factors limiting the rate of living-related kidney donation to children in an inner city setting. Pediatr Transplant 2001 Dec;5(6):419-24.

15. Butkus DE, Dottes AL, Meydrech EF, Barber WH. Effect of poverty and other socioeconomic variables on renal allograft survival. Transplantation 200127;72:261-6.

16. Fennell RS, Tucker C, Pedersen T. Demographic and medical predictors of medication compliance among ethnically different pediatric renal transplant patients. Pediatr Transplant 2001;5:343-8.

17. Tucker CM, Petersen S, Herman KC, Fennell RS, Bowling B, Pedersen T, Vosmik JR.Self-regulation predictors of medication adherence among ethnically different pediatric patients with renal transplants. J Pediatr Psychol 2001;26:455-64.

18. Callender CO, Washington AW. Organ/tissue donation the problem! Education the solution: a review. J Natl Med Assoc 1997;89:689-93.

19. Callender CO, Miles PV, Hall MB. National MOTTEP: educating to prevent the need for transplantation. Minority Organ Tissue Transplant Education Program. Ethn Dis 2002 Winter;12:S1-34-7.

20. Ozminkowski RJ, White AJ, Hassol A, Murphy M.. 1998 What if socioeconomics made no difference?: access to a cadaver kidney transplant as an example. Med Care;36:1398-406.

21. Hauptman PJ, O'Connor KJ. 1997 Procurement and allocation of solid organs for transplantation. N Engl J Med;336:422-31.

22. Friedlander MM. The right to sell or buy a kidney: are we failing our patients? Lancet 2002;359:971-973.

23. Glover JJ, Moss AH. 1998 Rationing dialysis in the United States: possible implications of capitated systems. Adv Ren Replace Thert;5:341-349.

24. Nilstun T, Ohlsson R. 1995 Should health care be rationed by age? Scand J Soc Med;23:81-84.

25. Channel 4000, 1997 James Michener Dies at 90 Internet Broadcasting Systems, Inc.

26. Edvardsson VO, Kaiser BA, Polinsky MS, Baluarte HJ. 1995 Successful living-related renal transplantation in an adolescent with Down syndrome. Pediatr Nephrol;9:398-389.

27. Schneiderman LJ, Jecker NS, Jonsen AR. 1990 Medical futility: its meaning and ethical implications. Ann Intern Med 1990 Jun 15;112:949-954.

28.   Flynn CT. The diabetic on CAPD. in Diabetic Renal-Retinal Syndrome. Prevention and Management 1982 (EA Friedman, FA L'Esperance, Jr. eds) pp 321-330.

29.   Perinbasekar S, Brod-Miller C, Pal S, Mattana J. Predictors of survival in HIV-infected patients on hemodialysis. Am J Nephrol 1996;16:280-286.

30.   Crawford PW. Urban renal disease: reflections of an urban nephrologist. Semin Nephrol 20011;21:329-33.

31.   Williams DR. Black-White differences in blood pressure: the role of social factors. Ethn Dis 1992;2:126-41.

32.   Bashar M, Alcabes P, Rom WN, Condos R. Increased incidence of multidrug-resistant tuberculosis in diabetic patients on the Bellevue Chest Service, 1987 to 1997. Chest 2001;120:1514-9.

33.   Delano BG, Suresh U, Feldman J, Schneider D, Friedman EA. Dismal rehabilitation in predominantly type II diabetics on dialysis in Inner-City Brooklyn. Clin Nephrol 2000;54-94-104.

34.   Kim MT, Dennison CR, Hill MN, Bone LR, Levine DM. Relationship of alcohol and illicit drug use with high blood pressure care and control among urban hypertensive Black men. Ethn Dis 2000;10:175-83.

35.   Hill MN, Bone LR, Kim MT, Miller DJ, Dennison CR, Levine DM.. Barriers to hypertension care and control in young urban black man. Am J Hypertens. 1999;12(12 Pt 1-2):1268-9.

36.   Graham HL, Maslin J, Copello A, Birchwood M. Mueser K, McGovern D, Georgiou G. Drug and alcohol problems amongst individuals with severe mental helath problems in an inner city area of the UK. Soc Psychiatry Psychiatr Epidemiol 2001;36:448-55.

37.   Demmer C. Impact of improved treatments on perceptions about

HIV and safer sex among inner-city HIV-infected men and women. J Community Health. 2002;27:63-73.

38. Lucas GM, Gebo KA, Chaisson RE, Moore RD. Longitudinal assessment of the effects of drug and alcohol abuse on HIV-1 treatment outcomes in an urban clinic. AIDS 2002;16:767-74.

39. Friedman AS, Glassman K, Terras BA. Violent behavior as related to use of marijuana and other drugs .J Addict Dis 2001;20:49-72.

40. Reese LE, Vera EM Thompson K, Reyes R. A qualitative investigation of perceptions of violence risk factors in low-income African American children. J Clin Child Psychol 2001;30:161-71.

41. Leggat JE Jr, Orzol SM, Hulbert-Shearon TE, Golper TA, Jones CA, Held PJ, Port FK. 1998 Noncompliance in hemodialysis: predictors and survival analysis. Am J Kidney Dis;32:139-145.

42. Anderson RJ, Matthews C. 1981 Non-compliance: failure of the therapeutic partnership. Cardiovasc Med;2:464-470.

43. Greenstein S, Siegal B.1998 Compliance and noncompliance in patients with a functioning renal transplant: a multi center study. Transplanatation;66:1718-1726.

44. Sermon MD. 1996 The combative patient: ethical issues in patient selection for chronic dialysis. Seminars Dialysis 1996;9:56-60.

45. Lundin AP. 1996 Causes of noncompliance in dialysis patients. Dialysis & Transplant;24:174-176, 202.

46. Procci WR. 1981 Psychological factors associated with severe abuse of the hemodialysis diet. Gen Hosp Psychiat;3:111-118.

47. Mid Atlantic Renal Coalition. Working with noncompliant and abusive patients. End-Stage Renal Disease network 5, Midlothian, Virginia, February 1994.

48.   Ifudu O, Dawood M, Homel P, Friedman EA. 1998 Excess morbidity in patients starting uremia therapy without prior care by a nephrologist. Am J Kidney Dis;28:841-845.

49.   McGuffin P, Murray RM, Reveley AM.1987 Genetic influence on the psychoses. Br Med Bull;43:531-536.

50.   Reich T. Listening With the Third Ear : The Inner Experience of a Psychoanalyst. Farrar, Straus & Giroux, Inc., New York. 1983.

51.   Sussman B, Spinal A.1997 Risky business: managing dangerous dialysis patients. Seminars Dialysis;10:282-285.

52.   Orenlicher D.1991 Denying treatment to the noncompliant patient. JAMA;266:1579-1582.

53.   Miller RB. 1995 Treating the disruptive patient. Nephrology News & Issues;9:39-40.

54.   Bower JD.1995 The issue: the role of the professional in the management of noncompliant or problem dialysis patients; Dialysis & Transplant 24:173,196.

55.   Beauchamp TL, Childress JF. Principles of Biomedical Ethics, New York, NY, Oxford University Press,1994.

56.   Spital A. Ethical issues in living organ donation. 1998 Nephrology Ethics Forum. Amer J Kidney Dis;32:676-691.

57.   Freer J. How to perform an ethics consult. Ethics Committee Core Curriculum. Online Edition. UB Center for Clinical Ethics and Humanities in Health Care,http://wings.buffalo.edu/faculty/research/bioethics/man-case.html, 10/18/98.

58.   Jamrozik K, Kolybaba M. 1999 Are ethics committees retarding the improvement of health services in Australia? Med J Aust;170:26-28.

59.   Chandna SM, Schulz J, Lawrence C, Greenwood RN, Farrington K. 1999 BMJ Jan 23;318(7178):217-223. Is there a rationale for rationing chronic dialysis? A hospital based cohort study of factors affecting survival and morbidity.

60.   Payne SK, Taylor RM. 1997 Semin Neurol;17:257-263. The persistent vegetative state and anencephaly: problematic paradigms for discussing futility and rationing.

61.   Klapheke MM. 1999 The role of the psychiatrist in organ transplantation. Bull Menninger Clin Winter;63:13-39.

62.   Corley MC, Westerberg N, Elswick RK Jr, Connell D, Neil J, Sneed G, Witcher V.1998 Rationing organs using psychosocial and lifestyle criteria. Res Nurs Health;21(4):327-337.

Has HAART Slowed the Epidemic of Human Immunodeficiency Virus-Associated Nephropathy (HIVAN)?
T.K. Sreepada Rao

Introduction

The identification of a new disease Acquired immunodeficiency syndrome (AIDS) in 1980-81, has had an unprecedented impact throughout the world, on the economic, social, ethical, and legal aspects of medical practice. But most importantly from a scientific perspective, major and rapid breakthroughs have occurred in the understanding of pathogenesis (molecular basis) of viral diseases in general, in the diagnostic techniques (serologic and viral markers) to monitor the progress/arrest of infection, and in the development of several classes of antiviral drugs for their treatment. In 1983-84, an unusual form of glomerular disease characterized by focal and segmental glomerulosclerosis (FSGS), rapid progression to end stage renal disease (ESRD) along with a high patient mortality, was described in patients with AIDS [1] Subsequently, when the causative agent Human immunodeficiency virus (HIV) was identified, the renal disease was referred to as HIV associated nephropathy (HIVAN). The disease has been extensively studied and reported by investigators both in the US and elsewhere. HIVAN was the fourth leading cause of ESRD in the US in Black men between the ages of 25 and 45 [2]. In 1985, the introduction of first antiretroviral drug Zidovudine (AZT), in the US a nucleoside reverse transcriptase inhibitor (NRTI);beneficially altered the natural history of HIV disease. In the subsequent years, several other classes of drugs; non-nucleoside reverse transcriptase inhibitors (NNRTI), protease inhibitors (PI), and others have revolutionized the modern management of patients with HIV infection. The term highly active antiretroviral therapy (HAART) was coined in 1995 to describe the effectiveness of combination of these antiretroviral drugs in suppressing/arresting HIV infection. In 1998, a dramatic 40% decline in AIDS related deaths attributable to HAART was reported. AIDS, which was the leading cause of death in men between the ages of 25 and 45 in the early 90's in the, has now dropped down to 5th leading cause.

This communication examines the question; has HAART impacted the epidemic of HIVAN?. What follows is a brief narration of the history of AIDS, milestones in the contributions of Kings County Hospital (KCH) and Downstate Medical Center (DMC) in the evolution of renal disease in AIDS. This is followed by a description of renal syndromes in HIV, and an analysis of the incidence and prevalence of both acute and irreversible renal failure in HIV patients prior to and after the introduction of HAART

Brief history of AIDS & kidney disease

In February 1980, the occurrence of PCP pneumonia & Kaposi's Sarcoma in otherwise healthy gay men at UCLA medical center, and subsequently in San Francisco, lead to the description of a new acquired immune deficiency disorder. A chronology of milestones in the evolution of this new disease AIDS, from its identification in 1980 to subsequent progress in the ensuing 20 years in the isolation of causative virus, introduction of diagnostic markers, various drug treatment regimen, and the current status of HIV disease in the US, are listed in Table I [3-5]. One can appreciate the rapid advancements in all aspects of HIV disease, and the anticipation is that in the coming years, through the use of refined and effective vaccines, HIV infection can be totally prevented and possibly eradicated. In 1983, the finding of a fulminant form of focal and segmental glomerulosclerosis (FSGS) in a young woman who presented with nephritic syndrome and esophageal candidiasis, and subsequently in a few more patients with similar renal manifestations, by workers in KCH in Brooklyn, NY, lead to the identification of an unusual form of AIDS associated nephropathy (AAN) [1]. The contributions of KCH/DMC in the evolution of renal disease in HIV from initial description to management of patients with HIVAN are shown in Table II. Pertinent to note are that these two urban centers have been in the forefront in describing the spectrum of renal disorders and managing HIV patients with ESRD.

Renal disorders in HIV patients

Renal complications in HIV disease, listed in detail in Table III, can be categorized into four broad groups:
1.   Co-incidental renal disorders.
2.   HIV associated glomerular diseases.
3.   Intrinsic renal disorders occurring in patients with prior HIV infection.
4.   HIHV infection developing in patients undergoing renal replacement therapy (RRP); maintenance dialysis (MD), and/or renal transplantation (RT).

With about two decades of experience, large body of data available todate provides us an opportunity to reterospectively examine the impact of HAART on these various renal syndromes in patients with HIV disease.

The most prominent co-incidental renal disorder pertinent to this communication, and encountered often in AIDS patients is a spectrum of acute renal failure (ARF) syndromes, primarily acute tubular necrosis (ATN). ARF in most clinical setting is associated with a high mortality, and in AIDS patients, its occurrence further worsens an already dim prognosis. ATN is a consequence of ischemic and toxic injury to kidneys in patients with AIDS suffering from multiple infections with hemodynamic/respiratory compromise who may also receive nephotoxic agents. Detailed discussions of ARF in HIV disease can be found in several recent reviews [6-8].

The spectrum of ATN in HIV patients varies from mild asymptomatic elevations in serum creatinine (Scr) concentrations to life threatening uremia requiring dialysis support and associated with a very high patient mortality. Therefore, in all of our studies dealing with ARF, we have included only the most severe forms namely patients with a Scr of 6 mg/dl or higher, and those requiring dialysis support. In Table IV, the annual incidence of ARF from 1983 to 2001 at KCH, in all hospitalized patients, and in those with HIV infection is tabulated.

Since 1995, a dramatic decline in the incidence of ARF in HIV patients has occurred. Between the years 1986-89, the annual incidence of severe ARF (those who needed dialysis support) in the hospitalized AIDS patients was 2%, which decreased to 1% between 1990-93, and has further declined to <0.5% in the years 1994-2001. While the reasons for these declines are unclear, it is logical to assume that the overall improvements in the care of

AIDS patients in general, and the use of HAART which has had a dramatic impact on AIDS related morbidity and mortality, may be responsible for this improvement.

HIV associated nephropathy (HIVAN)

Although a variety of glomerular lesions such as minimal change disease, membranous GN, Membrano-proliferative GN, immune complex GN, IgA nephropathy and others have been reported in HIV patients, we believe that the term HIVAN should be limited to those subjects in whom the histologic lesion in the kidney reveals FSGS [1-12]. H IVAN is most common in young black men, and although intravenous needle sharing drug abusers constitute the largest single group, the disease seen in patients irrespective of the mode of HIV infection, and also in children born to infected mothers.

The disease usually manifests as heavy proteinuria with the nephritic syndrome (generalized edema, hypoalbuminemia, with or without hyperlipidemia), accompanied by either a normal creatinine clearance (Ccr), or varying degrees of azotemia. Patients with HIVAN may also present with severe renal failure on their initial visit to the hospital. Occasionally, early features include hematuria, with non-nephrotic range proteinuria, along with normal or impaired Ccr. The majority of patients are normotensive, and continue to be so despite progression to irreversible uremia, an unusual finding in young black patients with ESRD. Investigations fails to detect other known causes of nephritic syndrome such as collagen vascular disease. HIVAN is generally considered to be a late manifestation of viral infection because studies reveal a severe depletion in the absolute number of circulating DC4 cells, along with high levels of plasma viral load [2]. Ultrasound examination reveals enlarged and markedly echogenic kidneys despite severe renal insufficiency.

The typical renal histologic lesion of HIVAN consists of collapsing form of FSGS, with intraglomerular deposition of IgM and C3, in association with tubulo-interstitial changes. The light microscopic features of HIV associated FSGS is also characterized by hyperplastic visceral epithelial cells with coarse cytoplasmic vacuoles, and protein absorption droplets in one or more lobules. There is a greater and widespread collapse of the underlying capillary walls, with obliteration of the lumen which are filled with lipid containing monocytes (foam cells). The most striking pathological features are seen in the renal tubules and alterations include severe tubular degenerataive changes, tubular microectasia commonly referred to as "microcystic dilatation", and the lumen is filled with pale staining protenaceous casts. There is a notable absence of interstitial infiltrates, interstitial fibrosis, and arteriolosclerotic changes of hypertension.

Under immunofluorescence microscopy, typically, there is localization of IgM, C3, and C1q in a granular form in the sclerosed glomerular segments, other mesangial regions, and capillary walls. Attempts to localize HIV antigens jn these presumed immune complexes have been uniformly unsuccessful. Characteristic ultrastructural lesions considered by some as distinctive consist of multiple complex inclusions both in the nuclei and cytoplasm in a variety of cells, abundant tubuloreticular inclusions (TRI) in the vascular (glomerular, peritubular capillary, arterial and venular) endothelium, and interstitial cell cytoplasm. While these manifestations are not specific for HIVAN, their combined presence in renal biopsies showing FSGS is very characteristic.

A prominent clinical finding is the absence of high blood pressure in a majority of patients with HIVAN and uremia, while moderate to severe hypertension is typically present in >85% of patients with ESRD from other causes. One distinctive clinical feature is the malignant nature of the syndrome and the rapidity with which renal functional deterioration occurs in HIVAN, in the absence of additional insult from anoxic injuries, hypovolemia, and nephrotoxic agents. In most large series, from the onset of proteinuria, ESRD has developed in 4-6 months, although wide variations in renal progression has been observed. Some have speculated that HIV infection of kidneys per se is responsible, and the HIVAN is a unique disease of combined glomerular, tubular and interstitial lesions. Cohen and co workers have provided objective evidence of a direct viral invasion of the kidneys to support this contention [13].

The pathogenesis of HIVAN is complex and involves an interplay of viral infection of kidney cells, dysregulated cytokine system, environmental and genetic factors. Demonstration of focal and segmental sclerosing glomerular lesions in Rhesus monkeys infected with the Simian immunodeficiency virus, and in cats infected with Feline immunodeficiency virus strengthen the role or viral infection of kidney cells. Recent demonstration of infection of endothelial, mesangial and epithelial cells by HIV provides additional evidence for the direct role of virus in HIVAN. The development of a transgenic mouse model using only non infectious component of HIV-1 proviral DNA, which develop proteinuria, azotemia, and FSGS suggests a major role for HIV proteins in the pathogeneseis [14]. The expression of HIV genes in transgenic mice may be responsible for enhanced mesangial accumulation of extracellular matrix protein, with the resulting pathology resembling human HIV associated FSGS.

Therapeutic agents which attempts to counteract these pathogenetic mechanisms and have shown beneficial results in patients with HIVAN include AZT, prednisone, Angiotensin converting enzyme inhibitors (ACEI), and HAART [15-20]. In the early years, AZT was the only antiretroviral agent in widespread use, and reported results in HIVAN were less than optimistic. Currently, AZT is used always in combination with other antiretroviral agents in HIV patients.

Prednisone therapy in selected patients with HIVAN has shown remarkable results including in some, recovery of sufficient renal function to withhold dialysis support. Because of potential risks of corticosteroids in precipitating or aggravating conventional and opportunistic infections in already immunosuppressed HIV patients, it is prudent that prednisone therapy not only be used with caution in a few selected patients, but also limit the duration of administration.

Now in the era of HAART, isolated reports are beginning to document its beneficial effects on the natural history of HIVAN. Currently, the deployment of HAART, a standard of care in patients with HIV disease without kidney disease has lead to dramatic declines in morbidity and mortality. It is therefore logical to assess the impact of HAART on both the natural history of HIVAN, and also survival in HIV patients with ESRD treated by RRT. Since it is unethical to withhold anti retroviral therapy in the present era, no doubt blind controlled studies exist to answer this question with certainty. WE have to rely on historic controls, to assess the impact of HAART by indirectly analyzing published data of the incidence/prevalence rates of new onset ESRD in patients with HIV.

One remarkable example of the impact of HAART is the experiences observed and reported in children with HIVAN and ESRD. The implementation of widespread screening of pregnant women for HIV infection, diagnosis of infected infants at birth, and institution of early and effective antiretroviral treatment has resulted in almost complete disappearance of HIVAN in children in the last decade.

The prevalence of HIV patients with ESRD in the US as recorded in the RSRDS are summarized in Tables V. Since 1993, in the US, there has been a progressive increase in the number of patients with ESRD from all causes, as well as those with HIV infection. This increase in HIV patients with ESRD can be attributed to improvement in survival most likely as a result of widespread use of HAART in those treated by MD. In Table VI, annual incidence of new onset ESRD in HIV patients is listed. it is obvious that there has been a progressive decrease in the incidence from 1995 to 1999. The incidence of ESRD in H IV patients in NY State are tabulated in Tables VII. While the data is incomplete, it is obvious that there has been a dramatic decline in ESRD in HIV patients in the years 1999 and 2000 (2.5% and 2% respectively) as compared to 8% during the years 1986-95.

Could this decrease be due to HAART?. The issue is unclear. Listed in Table VIII, is the data from KCH, Brooklyn, NY of all new ESRD patients (all causes), and those with HIV infection from 1984 to 2000, broken down into three years intervals. At the height of AIDS epidemic, HIVAN accounted for 31% of all ESRD patients starting MH at KCH, which has been progressively declining over the recent years. The incidence has been steady at 16% over the past 6 years. From these data, we can only conclude that the trend in the incidence of ESRD secondary to HIVAN at KCH while certainly not increasing, seems to show a declining trend. Once agin, the reasons are unclear, but speculations are that the overall improvement in the care of HIV infected patients including HAART may be responsible for these decline both in Brooklyn and NY State and in the US.

Unrelated renal disease and HIV

Current estimates are that there are more than a million individuals who are infected with the virus in the U.S., and are seropositive for HIV. It is logical to expect that some of these patients will develop renal disease secondary to other etiologies such as diabetes mellitus, polycystic kidneys, systemic lupus erythematosus, and other primary disorders. Although no data is available, it is possible that with marked improvement in survival as a result of HAART, it is possible that in the coming years, we may actually see an increase in the number of HIV patients with ESRD from disorders unrelated to HIV. On the other hand, ESRD patients who are receiving RRT (either MD or RT) are unlikely to acquire new HIV infection from blood transfusion or through renal allograft. Mandatory screening of all potential blood and tissue donors and refinements in diagnostic procedures to identify seronegative persons, has practically eliminated such modes of viral transmission.

In summary, HAART has had a great impact in improving the survival in HIV patients without kidney disease, and also in those with ESRD undergoing MD. Because of lack of controlled studies, while it is difficult to asses with certainty the effects of HAART on a variety of renal syndromes encountered in HIV patients, it is fair to say that the incidence of severe ARF has definitely declined. The incidence of HIVAN in the US and NY State shows a definite downward trend. In Brooklyn, NY while the incidence of HIVAN is clearly not increasing, it is possible it may be declining as well.

T.K. Sreepada Rao, M.D., F.A.C.P.
Renal Disease Division
Department of Medicine
SUNY Downstate Medical Center
Brooklyn, New York

References

1.   Winston JA, Burns GC, Klotman PE. THe human immunodeficiency virus (HIV) epidemic and HIV-associated nephropathy. Semin Nephrol 1998;18:373-7.

2.   Rao TKS, Filippone EJ, Nicastri AD, et al. Associated focal and segmental glomerulosclerosis in the acquired immunodeficiency syndrome. N Engl J Med 1984;310:669-73.

3.   Gold J, Dwyer J. A short history of AIDS. The Med J of Aust 1994;160:251-2.

5.   Timeline of the AIDS epidemic. http://www.alpa.org/apla/ed/ TIMELINE.HTM.

6.   AIDS History Project, Chronology of AIDS in San Francisco. http: //www.library.ucsf.edu

7.   Rao TKS, Friedman EA. Outcome of severe acute renal failure in patients with the acquired immunodeficiency syndrome. Am J Kidney Dis 1995;25(3):390-398.

8.   Rao TKS. Renal complications in HIV disease. Med Clin N Amer 1996;80(6):1437-1451.

9.   Rao TKS. Human immunodeficiency virus infection and Renal failure in "Infectious Disease Clinics of North America", Pien, F. Editor, Sept, 2001, W.B. Saunders, Philadelphia, PA.

10.   Rao TKS, Friedman EA, Nicastri AD. The types of renal disease in the acquired immunodeficiency syndrome. N Engl J Med 1987;316: 1062-68.

11.   Humphreys MH. Human immunodeficiency virus-associated glomerulosclerosis. Kidney Int 1995;48:311-320.

12.   D'Agati V, Appel GB. HIV infection and the kidney. J Amer Soc Nephrol 1997;8(1):138-152.

13.   Rao TKS, Chander P. Secondary focal segmental glomerulosclerosis, in "Comprehensive Nephrology", Johnson RJ, Feehaly J, Editors, Pages 23.1-23.10, Mosby International, London, UK, 1999.

14.   Cohen AH. Renal pathology of HIV associated nephropathy, in: Kimmel PL, Berns JS, editors. Renal and urologic aspects of HIV

infection, New York, Churchill Livingstone, 1995, p 155-180.

15. Bruggeman LA, Dickman S, Meng C, et al. Nephropathy in human immunodeficiency virus-1 transgenic mice is due to transgene expression. J Clin Invest 1997;100(1):84-92.

16. Ifudu O, Rao TKS, Tan CC, Fleischman H, Chirgwin K. Friedman EA. Zidovudine is beneficial in human immunodeficiency virus associated nephropathy. Am J Nephrol 1995;15:217-221.

17. Smith MC, Austen JL, Carey JT, et al. Prednisone improves renal function and proteinuria in human immunodeficiency virus-associated nephropathy. Am J Med 1996;101:41-8.

18. Burns GC, Paul SK, Toth IR, Sivak SL. Effect of angiotensin-converting enzyme inhibition in HIV-associated nephropathy. J Amer Soc Nephrol. 1997;8:1140-6.

19. Viani RM, Dankner WM, Muelenaer PA, Spector SA. Resolution of HIV-1-associated nephritic syndrome with highly active antiretrovital therapy delivered by gastrostomy tube. Pediatrics 1999;104(6):1394-96.

20. Wali RK, Drachenberg CI, Papadimitriou JC, et al. HIV-1-associated nephropathy and response to highly-active antiretrovital therapy. Lancet 1998;352:783-4.

21. Dellow E, Unwin R, Miller R, et al. Protease inhibitor therapy for HIV infection: the effect on HIV-associated nephritic syndrome. Nephrol Dial Transplant 1999;14:744-7.

11. Chapelon C, Raguin G, De Gennes C. Renal insufficiency with nebulised pentamidine. Lancet 1989;1:1045-6.

12. Sattler FR, Cowan R, Nielsen M, Ruskin J. Trimethoprim Sulphamethaxazole compared with Pentamidine for the treatment of pnemocystis carinii pneumonia in the Acquired immunodeficiency syndrome. Ann Int Med 1988;109:280-7.

13. Myre SA, McCann J, First MR, Cluxton Jr. RJ. Effect of Trimethoprim on serum creatinine in healthy and chronic renal failure volunteers. Ther Drug Monit 1987;9(2):161-5.

14. Nissenson AR, Wilson C, Holazo A. Pharmacokinetics of intravenous Trimethoprim Sulphamethaxazole during hemodialysis. Amer J Nephrol. 1987;7(4):270-4.

15. Siber GR, Gorham CC, Ericson JF, Smith AL. Pharmacokinetics of intravenous trimethoprim-sulfamethoxazole in children and adults

with normal and impaired renal function. Rev Infect Dis 1982;4: 566-78.

16. Raymond J. Amphotericin nephrotoxicity. Amer Fam Pract 1988;38: 199-203.

17. Branch RA. Prevention of amphotericin-B induced renal impairment. Arch Int Med 1988;148:2389-94.

18. Cacoub P, Deray G, Baumelou A, LeHoang P, Rozenbaum W, Gentilini M, Soubrie C. Rousselie F, Jacobs C. Acute renal failure induced by foscarnet: 4 cases. Clin Nephrol 1988;29(6):315-8.

19. Deray G, Martinex F, Katlama C, Levaltier B, Beaufils H, Rozenheim M, Baumelou A, Dohin E, Gentilini M. Foscarnet nephrotoxicity: mechanism, incidence, and prevention. Amer J Nephrol 1989;9(4): 316-21.

20. Rosenberg SA, Lotze MT, Mule JJ. New approaches to the immunotherapy of cancer using Interleukin-2. Ann Int Med 1988;108:853-64.

21. Christiansen NP, Skubitz KM, Nath K, Ochoa A, Kennedy BJ. Nephrotoxicity of continuous intravenous infusion of recombinant Interleukin-2. Amer J Med 1988;84:1072-5.

Table I

A snap shot of the History of Aids

1980 Michael Gottlieb at UCLA reports PCP pneumonia & Kaposi's Sarcoma in healthy gay men

1981 CDC officially recognizes a new disease.

1982 CDC officially names the disease AIDS (replacing Gay cancer, gay related immune deficiency).

1983-84 Isolation of virus. Luc Montagne from Pasteur Institute in Paris names the virus LAV (Lymphadenopathy associated virus). Robert Gallo at NIH calls it HTLV III (Human T lyphotropic virus III).

1985 Elisa assay for detection of antibodies to virus in the blood is introduced for diagnosis of infected patients.

1986 CDC proposes a classification of AIDS.

1987 First antiretroviral drug Azidothymidine (AZT), a nucleoside reverse transcriptase inhibitor (NRTI) is deployed for treatment.

1989 NIVp24 antigen assay deployed in diagnosing acute infection.

1991 ddI (Diadenosine), second antiretroviral drug approved.

1995 Saquinavir, a protease inhibitor (PI) introduced for treatment.

1996 Nevirapine, a nonnucleoside reverse transcriptase inhibitor (NNRTI) is approved.

1992-99 4 more NRTI's, 2 more NNRTI's, and 5 more PI's are approved.

1995 The term HAART (Highly active antiretroviral therapy) is introduced.

1996 HIV viral load assay introduce din clinical practice to determine the severity of infection, and to follow the efficacy of HAART.

1998 First dramatic decline in deaths from AIDS reported.

Table II

A snap shot of KCH-DMC contribution to Kidney Disease in HIV

1983 – 84 FSGS in a young woman with esophageal candidiasis and nephritic syndrome, and in 6 more patients, leads to identification of AIDS associated nephropathy.

1985 Guidelines for hemodialysis delivery developed. Dismal prognosis in AIDS patients with ESRD who undergo hemodialysis is reported.

1985 – 87 Controversy regarding the existence of AAN resolved.

1987 Renal manifestations in AIDS patients described in more detail, and classification proposed.

1988 Description of nephropathy as initial manifestation in some asymptomatic HIV patients.

1990 Renal disease in HIV patients is included in major renal text books.

1995 Results of AZT therapy in AAN reported.

1995 Use of Erythropoietin in ESRD patients with HIV reported.

1995 Detailed review of ARF in AIDS patients reported.

1997 Improved survival in ESRD patients with HIV infection undergoing maintenance hemodialysis reported.

Table III

Renal disorders in patients with HIV

<u>Incidental Renal disease and HIV infection:</u>

Various forms of potentially reversible acute renal failure.

<u>I. Specific? renal disease: HIV Associated Nephropathy:</u>

a. Focal and segmental glomerulosclerosis.

b. Other forms of glomerulopathy.

<u>II. Unrelated renal disease in HIV infected patients:</u>

a. Heroin associated nephropathy.

b. Diabetic nephropathy, polycystic kidney disease etc.

c. Obstructive nephropathy.

<u>V. HIV infection in ESRD patients receiving Renal Replacement Therapy:</u>

      1.   Maintenance dialysis patients acquiring HIV from contaminated blood transfusions, intravenous drug abuse, and sexual contacts.

      2.   Renal transplant recipients developing HIV infection through renal allograft, contaminated blood transfusions, intravenous drug abuse, and sexual contacts.

Table IV

Acute Renal Failure & HIV Disease

<u>Annual Incidence of ARF at KCH</u>

YEARS	**ARF (All Causes)**	**ARF HIV Pts**	**INCIDENCE/ Non-HIV HIV**	**YEAR**
1983 – 1986	162	47	29	12
1987 – 1990	198	69	32	17
1991 – 1994	149	49	25	12
1995 – 1998	130	21	28	5
1999 – 2001	84	9	25	3

Table V

Annual Prevalence of ESRD in HIV patients in the US**

YEAR	All ESRD Patients	HIV Pts With ESRD	% of Total
1993	160,426	297	0.1%
1994	177,660	586	0.3%
1995	234,296	950	0.4%
1996	255,573	1358	0.6%
1997	305,876	2646	0.8%
1998	398,158	3959	0.94%
1999	406,310	4271	1.05%

Note the annual increase in number of patients with HIV and ESRD
Attributable to improved survival
**Source: USRDS

Table VI

Annual Incidence of ESRD in HIV patients in the US**

YEAR	All New ESRD Pts	HIV Pts With ESRD	% of Total
1995	43,286	648	1.50%
1996	68,869	774	1.12%
1997	74,465	950	0.96%
1998	79,135	738	0.93%
1999	85,343	696	0.81%

Note the annual decrease in number of patients with HIV and ESRD Attributable to HAART?

**Source : USRDS

Table VII

Incidence of ESRD in HIV in NY State

YEAR	All New ESRD Pts	HIV Pts With ESRD	% of Total
1986-95*	15,000	1174	8.0%
1999**	6,291	155	2.5%
2000**	6,563	130	2.0%

Table VIII

Incidence of ESRD in HIV at KCH

YEARS	All New ESRD Pts	HIV Pts With ESRD	% of Total
1984-86	290	31	9.31
1987-89	258	56	19.0
1990-92	242	76	31.0
1993-95	294	60	20.4
1996-98	206	33	16.5
1999-01	217	36	16.0

Note the dramatic decline after 1992
and the trend for further drop since 1995

CAPD or Hemodialysis: Which for the Urban Poor?

Barbara G. Delano, MD, MPH,

Introduction

While a successful transplant is the optimum treatment for end stage renal disease, the great majority of patient undergo hemodialysis. The factors involved in the choice of modality are not well understood. It is clear however, that a patient cannot choose a therapy unless he or she is aware of it. According to the 2001 United States Renal Data System (USRDS), in 1999, the vast majority of dialysis patients were on in-center hemodialysis (90%) with less than 1 percent of patients on home hemodialysis and 9 percent receiving some form of peritoneal dialysis [1]. There are also differences in treatment modality according to race, with black patients less likely to undergo peritoneal dialysis. Figure 1 shows the percentage of white and black patients on the various modes of dialytic therapy in 1999. While the percentage of black patients who perform home hemodialysis is proportionally higher than that of all black son dialysis, these numbers are very small. What is clear is that black patients are less likely than whites to either select or be offered peritoneal dialysis. In 1999, 71% of new peritoneal dialysis patients were white and 19% were black [1]. In this paper, we will discuss which if any therapy is better suited to the urban poor.

In discussing dialytic therapies, my biases are the following: 1) Home hemodialysis offers the best survival and rehabilitation and is possible in the inner city: 2) Patients undergoing hemodialysis and peritoneal dialysis have equivalent survival according to which papers you read: 3) Black patienets have superior survival than their white counterparts in both hemodialysis and peritoneal dialysis, despite having a lower socioeconomic standard.

Home hemodialysis offers the best survival and rehabilitation

Home hemodialysis while currently performed by less than 1 percent of dialysis patients in the United States has been shown to have superior survival and rehabilitation when compared to in-center dialysis. Woods and coworkers, using the USRDS special case mix severity standard analysis file, collected data on 3102 in-center and 70 home hemodialysis patients. Home hemodialysis patients were significantly younger, mean age 49 vs. 59 years, and less likely than in-center patients to have diabetes mellitus listed as a cause of their renal failure (14% versus 30%). They were also more likely to be white and male, although this did not reach statistical significance. Unadjusted, there was a significant survival benefit of performing hemodialysis at home compared to in-center, (RR 0.37, 95% confidence interval 0.22-0.60). Even after correcting for age, diabetes and co-morbid conditions, using Cox proportional hazards' technique, the patients on home dialysis were still 42% times less likely to die than their in-center counterparts for the four-year period studied (RR 0.58, 95% confidence interval 0.35l-0.95) [2].

Mailloux, et al, studied patient outcomes during a 24-year period in a more middle class setting. They found a 20-year survival estimate of 35% for patients on home hemodialysis while in-center patients had a 5 percent estimate for the same time period [3]. Home hemodialysis is also possible among the rural poor. In 1989, Rubin, Hsu and Bower reported on their experience performing home hemodialysis in rural Alabama, Arkansas and Mississippi. In that area, ESRD Network 18, at that time, there were proportionally more black patients on dialysis than in the nation as a whole, 53% vs. 29%. The median technique survival for home hemodialysis was 7.5 years, compared to a median technique survival of 1.9 years for patients on chronic ambulatory peritoneal dialysis [4]. That program still has 50 mostly indigent, (85% on Medicaid), patients on home hemodialysis. (Personnel communication, Dr. John Bower).

Delano has shown that home hemodialysis can be successfully performed in the inner-city. The mean survival of 133 middle class patients in that program was no different from that of 71 patients classified as indigent [5].

Onyekachi Ifudu

Peritoneal dialysis and in-center dialysis offer equivalent survival

The debate as to whether or not peritoneal dialysis is an equally effective therapy as hemodialysis can never be satisfactorily answered unless one performs a study randomly assigning patients to both therapies and following them prospectively. This is not practical and of course, unethical. Thus, we have to interpret the available observational studies. A sentinel paper addressing this issue was published by Bloembergen, et al. This was an as-treated analysis of more than 170,000 prevalent patients on January first of 1987-1989. Patients were followed for one year and censored at transplantation. Patients undergoing peritoneal dialysis were overall 19% more likely to die than those treated in-center (RR 1.19, P < 0.001). This risk however was insignificant for patients younger than age 55, but worse for patients with diabetes mellitus (RR 1.38, P < 0.001) [6].

By contrast, data from the Canadian Organ Replacement Registry (CORR) studying incident patients, who started renal replacement therapy between 1990-1994, found that patients on peritoneal dialysis were less likely to die than those on hemodialysis (RR 0.73, 95% CI 0.68-0.78). This survival advantage was concentrated in the first two years of therapy and by four years the survival was equal in both groups [7].

Collins and coworkers attempting to clarify the United States comparative mortality rates, designed a study using incident patients, censored two months after a modality change and at time of transplantation. They used an interval Poisson and a Cox regression. Treatment with peritoneal dialysis was associated with a significantly lower death risk, with the exception of diabetic women older than age 55 [8].

Shinzato and co-workers evaluated survival of dialysis patients in Japan since 1966. They surveyed virtually every dialysis facility and had a response rate approaching 100%. One, five and ten year patient survival were 95%, 67%, and 49% for peritoneal dialysis and 89%, 60% and 39% for hemodialysis [9].

It is difficult to evaluate these data since the various studies have methological differences. I believe that based on the current literature, in advising an individual patient about dialytic therapy, survival differences are not as important as life style choices.

Blacks survive better of all dialytic therapies (despite having a lower socioeconomic status)

In the United States, black patients have better survival on both hemodialysis and peritoneal dialysis. Table I shows the adjusted death rates for Whites and Blacks for peritoneal and hemodialysis as recorded by the USRDS. The survival advantage for black patients is evident in both the first and second year of dialysis treatment [1]. Pei, Greenwood, Cherry and Wu examined clinical data on four different ethnic groups undergoing dialytic therapy in Toronto. After controlling for co-morbidity and demographic factors, they found that the risk of death in white patients was significantly increased when compared with Southeast Asians, South Asians and black patients. Relative risk of death for the respective groups was 1.63, 1.36, 1.34, and 1 [10].

Does the superior dialysis survival seen by black patient also occur in the "inner city?" Tanna, Vonesh and Korbet retrospectively evaluated 432 patients (78% black) on both peritoneal and hemodiaylsis in an urban setting. Blacks compromised 70% of the peritoneal and 84% of the hemodialysis patients. Overall, peritoneal dialysis survival was superior to hemodialysis. Black patients especially did better on peritoneal dialysis versus hemodialysis with a one, two and five-year survival rate of 92%, 80%, and 52% for peritoneal dialysis, compared to 88%, 74%, and 40% on hemodialysis, P=0.09 [11].

In another study of incident patients in a large urban peritoneal dialysis unit with 61% Black and 12% Hispanic patients, the authors tried to identify possible ethnic differences in survival. This group has provided peritoneal dialysis for more than 18 years in this urban setting. The relative risk of mortality for white patients compared to blacks was 2.35. They conclude that peritoneal dialysis should be considered a viable option for black patients beginning treatment for end stage renal disease [12].

Stivelman, et al evaluated the survival rates over three years in a large inner-city dialysis unit in which 94% of the patients were Black and 50% had an annual income of less than $7,000. They calculated standardized mortality ratios (SMR) using USRDS data for the expected value. For each year studied, they had a significantly lower SMR than the United States average. The authors conclude that despite economic hardship, patients given good dialysis and adequate support can do better than the national survival average on renal replacement therapy [13].

If black patients do well on peritoneal dialysis, but are under represented in the modality, it may be instructive to examine how patients select a treatment. There is data to show that patients who have pre-end stage renal disease education are more likely to select peritoneal dialysis [14,15]. Ifudu and coworkers reported that patients who were Black, Hispanic, and older were more likely to have delayed referral to a nephrologist [16]. Presumable, patients referred to a nephrologists would be more likely to undergo education.

In a recent study of factors associated with selection of home therapies in six dialysis units in inner-city Brooklyn, we found that only 46% of all patients had seen a nephrologist before starting renal replacement therapy and 13% had not seen any physician, but arrived in the local emergency rooms uremic and requiring urgent dialysis[17]. Winklemayer using a regression analysis found that socioeconomic status, but not black race was associated with late referral to a nephrologist [18]. This same group subsequently found that black race (odds ration 0.56) and lower socioeconomic status (odds ration 0.68), but not late referrals were reasons for patients not receiving peritoneal dialysis [19].

In conclusion, I believe that urban inner city residents who are economically disadvantaged, as well as middle class patients, can perform any dialysis successfully. As home dialysis (especially home hemodialysis) offers better survival and rehabilitation as well as improved quality of life, hopefully patients will select this. Newer technology that makes dialysis at home easier may make these therapies more attractive. Patients awaiting transplantation, or not medically suitable for one, should be encouraged to perform one of the home therapies.

Barbara Delano, M.D., M.P.H.
Renal Disease Division
Department of Medicine
SUNY Downstate Medical Center
Brooklyn, New York

References

1. U.S. Renal Data System: USRDS 2001 Annual Report. Bethesda, MD: The National Institute of Diabetes and Digestive and Kidney Diseases: March 2001.

2. Woods JD, Port FK, Stannard D, Blass CR, Held PJ. Comparison of mortality with home hemodialysis and center hemodialysis: A national study. Kidney Inter 1996;49:1464-1470.

3. Mailloux LU, Kapikian N, Napolitano B, et al. Home Hemodialysis: Patient outcomes duringa 24-year period of time from 1970 through 1993. Advances in Renal Replacement Therapy 1996;3:112-119.

4. Rubin J, Hsu H, Bower J. Survival on dialysis therapy: One center's experience. Am J Medical Sciences 1989;297:80-89.

5. Delano BG: Home Hemodialysis offers excellent survival. Advances in Renal Replacement Therapy 1996;3:102-111.

6. Bloemenbergen WE, Port FK, Mauger EA, Wolfe RA. A comparison of mortality between patients treated with hemodialysis and peritoneal dialysis. J Am Soc Nephrol 1995;6:177-183.

7. Fenton SA, Schaulbel DE, Desmeules M, et al. Hemodialysis versus peritoneal dialysis: A comparison of adjusted mortality rates. Am J Kidney Dis 1997;30-334-342.

8. Collins AJ, Hao Wenli, Xia H, et al: Mortality risk of peritoneal dialysis and hemodialysis. Am J Kidney Dis 1999;34:1065-1074.

9. Shinzato T, Nakai S, Akiba T, et al. Report of the annual statistical survey of the Japanese Society for Dialysis Therapy in 1996. Kidney Int 1999;55:700-712.

10. Pei YP, Greenwood CM, Cherry AL, Wu, CC. Racial differences in survival of patients on dialysis. Kidney Int 2000;58:1293-1299.

11. Tanna MM, Vonesh EF, Korbet SM. Patients survival among incident peritoneal dialysis patients in an urban setting. Am J Kidney Dis 2000;36:1175-82.

12. Korbet SM, Shih D, Cline KN, Vonesh EF. Racial differences in survival in an urban peritoneal dialysis program. Am J Kidney Dis 1991;34:713-720.

13. Stivelman JC, Soucie JM, Hall ES, Macon EJ. Dialysis survival in a large inner-city facility: a comparison to national rates. J Am Soc Nephrol 1995;6:1256-61.

14. Levin A, Lewis M, Mortiboy P, et al. Multi disciplinary predialysis programs. Quantification of their impact on patients outcomes in two Canadian settings. Am J Kidney Dis 1997;29:533-540.

15. Schmidt RJ, Domino JR, Sorkin MI, Hobbs G. Early referral and its impact on emergent first dialysis, health care costs and outcome. Am J Kidney Dis 1998;32:278-283.

16. Ifudu O, Dawood M, Iofel Y, Valcourt JS, Friedman EA. Delayed referral of black, Hispanic and older patients with chronic renal failure. Am J Kidney Dis 1999;4:728-733.

17. Delano BG, Markell MS, Wolf F, Yuova S, Friedman EA, Salifu MO. Knowledge of home dialysis among satellite hemodialysis patients in the inner city. (Abs) Peritoneal Dial Intern 2002;22:S57.

18. Winkelmayer WC, Glynn RJ, Levin R. Owens WF, Avorn J. Determinants of delayed. Nephrologist referral in patients with chronic kidney disease. Am J Kidney Dis 2001;38:1178-1184.

19. Winkelmayer WC, Flyn RJ, Levin R, Owen W jr, Avorn J. Later referral and modality in end-stage renal disease. Kidney Int 2001;60: 1547-54.

Figure I

Percentage of Black and White patients undergoing in center hemodialysis, peritoneal dialysis and home hemodialysis in 1999

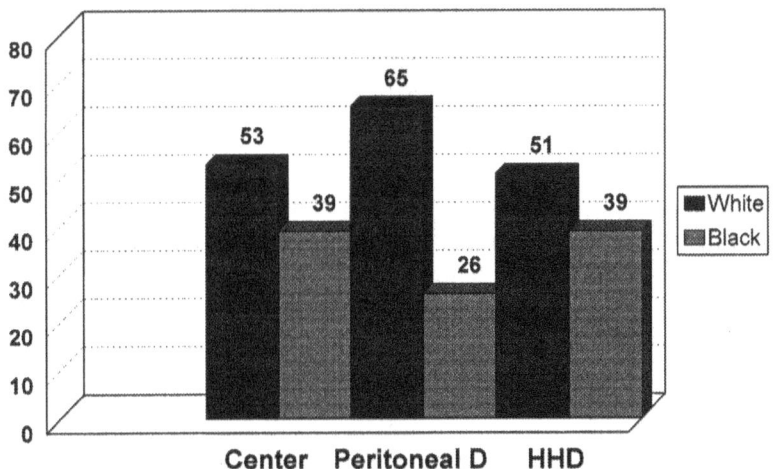

Gynecologic And Reproductive Issues In End-Stage Renal Disease

Iram Anees, M. D.

Introduction

Disturbances in menstrual cycle reduced libido are frequently found both in women with chronic renal failure and those who have reached end-stage renal disease (ESRD). The major menstrual abnormality in uremic women is anovulation, which in turn leads to infertility. Hyperprolactinemia, which is commonly found, may lead to impaired hypothalamic-pituitary function and contribute to sexual dysfunction and galactorrhea in these patients. Though bromocriptine corrects the hyperprolactinemia in these patients but usually does not restore normal menses, thereby suggesting that other mechanisms are also involved. Sexual dysfunction is reported in about 66-75% of women on dialysis in Amsterdam as compared to 14.7% of women in general Dutch population. Prevalence of sexual problems in renal replacement therapy population is extremely high, both in absolute percentage and in comparison to general population.

Uremic women with amenorrhea may be at increased risk of endometrial cancer due to unopposed proliferative effect of estrogen. These women should have gynecological evaluation at regular intervals. Women with ESRD having regular menses should be counseled about birth control. The chance of pregnancy in this setting is low but real. Maternal hypertension and increased proteinuria are the major maternal morbidities both in women with chronic renal failure and those on dialysis.

An accelerated loss of renal function is seen in women with a baseline serum creatinine of 2.0 mg/ dl or greater prior to or at the time of conception. Pregnancy does not seem to have an adverse effect on renal allograft survival or function if mother's serum creatinine is less than 1.5-2.0 mg/ dl.

54

Growth retardation and prematurity are seen commonly in infants born to women with chronic renal failure and those undergoing any kind of renal replacement therapy. Women's health issues like screening for gynecologic cancers and prescribing hormone replacement therapy is grossly neglected in women on dialysis. Hormone replacement therapy may reduce the risk of fracture in these women and improve overall lipid profile. A systematic study of this area is long overdue.

Scope of the Problem

Problems and abnormalities in sexual function are common in both men and women with chronic renal failure (1,2). Although the exact pathogenetic mechanisms for this sexual dysfunction are not entirely clear but it is speculated that it is mutifactorial in etiology and is primarily organic. Peripheral vascular disease, autonomic and peripheral neuropathy, uremic milieu, anemia, fatigue, stress and depression associated with chronic illness, and pharmacologic therapy all may contribute to genesis of this problem.

Menstrual abnormalities and sexual dysfunction in uremic women

Disturbances in menstrual cycle are frequently found not only in women with End-stage Renal Disease (ESRD) but in also those women with lesser degrees in chronic renal insufficiency. In the early 1980's most of the women who were receiving either hemodialysis (HD) or peritoneal dialysis (PD) were reported to be amenorrheic . The menstrual disturbances typically persisted even after initiation of maintenance dialytic therapy. In a small percentage of women, menorrhagia develops, sometimes leading to increased erythropoietin or transfusion requirements. Approximately 10% of women with ESRD were claimed to have regular menstrual cycles (3-5).

In marked contrast, Holley et al (6) in a study published in 1997 found that as many as 42% of women on dialysis (68% on HD and 32% on PD) reported having regular menstrual cycles when a cross sectional survey was done. The authors acknowledged the fact that the reason for this discrepancy in the older literature and their study was not clear, but speculated if the use of recombinant human erythropoietin and its possible effects on hypothalamic function might be contributory. Higher hematocrits and improved dialysis delivery may have a beneficial effect on hypothalamic pituitary function.

The major menstrual abnormality in uremic women is anovulation with affected patients being infertile (7-9). To comprehend the abnormalities in menstrual cycle or uremic women, one must understand the normal menstrual cycle, which is divided into a follicular or proliferative phase and a luteal or secretory phase. Normal follicular maturation and subsequent ovulation requires appropriately timed secretion of the pituitary gonadotrophins, follicle stimulating hormone (FSH) and uteinizing hormone (LH). FSH secretion exhibits negative feedback, with hormone levels falling as the plasma estrogen concentration falls (9). On the contrary, LH secretion is maximally suppressed by low levels of estrogen but exhibits positive feedback control in response to a rising and sustained elevation of estradiol. Therefore, high levels of estradiol in the late follicular phase trigger a surging elevation in LH secretion, which in turn causes a mature ovum to shed off causing ovulation to occur. Serum progesterone levels increase after ovulation as the follicle, which is now called corpus luteal or secretory phase.

Three different lines of evidence suggest that anovulatory cycles are the rule in uremic women (4,7,10). Firstly, endometrial biopsies show an absence of progestational effects. Secondly, at the expected time of ovulation, basal body temperature fails to rise in uremic women. Lastly, when measured biochemically, the preovulatory peak in LH and estradiol concentrations is frequently absent. Women with chronic renal failure commonly have increased serum prolactin levels, which appears to be autonomous in this setting as it is resistant to maneuvers designed to stimulate or inhibit its release. It has been suggested that the elevated prolactin levels may impair hypothalamic-pituitary function and contribute to sexual dysfunction and galactorrhea in uremic women. Though bromocriptine corrects the hyperprolactinemia in these patients but usually does not restore normal menses (4,5), thereby suggesting that other mechanisms are also involved.

The results of a recent sexual dysfunction questionnaire survey done in Amsterdam, Netherlands showed that in comparison to 15% women and 8.7% men in general Dutch population (n=591), about 75% and 62.9% patients on hemodilaysis, 66% and 69% on peritoneal dialysis (n=400), 44% and 48% with a well functioning renal transplant (n=300) (women and men respectively) complained of sexual dysfunction (11). The results of the simple questionnaire were sufficiently validated when 102 of 104 patients confirmed their responses in a subsequent structured interview by a sexologist. Only in male patients, was an association between the prevalence of a sexual problem and age found. This study reconfirms that prevalence of sexual problems in renal replacement therapy population is extremely high, both in absolute percentage and in comparison to general population.

Moreover, although renal transplant patients had significantly less sexual dysfunction as compared with the patients on either hemo or peritoneal dialysis but they still had markedly greater sexual dysfunction as compared to general population.Palmer et al (9) suggests that it may be desirable in at least some of the uremic amenorrheic women to administer a progestational agent during the final days of menstrual cycle for a few months in the year.

The idea is to reduce the enhanced risk of uterine cancer in these women with unopposed proliferative effect of estrogen on uterine endometrium by the progesterone. Furthermore, for the above-mentioned reason, a gynecologist should monitor these women closely. Women having regular menses on dialysis should be counseled about birth control as the chance of an unwanted and unexpected pregnancy, although small, is real. Lastly, estradiol therapy or bromocriptine therapy can be tried with variable success for treatment of reduced libido in uremic women. Adequate dialysis dose and target hematocrit of 33-36 shall be sought. Any culprit medications that may contribute to reduced libido shall be discontinued. Successful renal transplantation appears to be the most effective means of restoring normal sexual desire in women with chronic renal failure (2).

Pregnancy in Chronic Renal Insufficiency and End stage Renal Disease

An anovulation leads to infertility, the rate of pregnancy both in women with chronic renal failure and those on dialysis is substantially reduced.Conception rate in women on dialysis has been reported from anywhere between 0.3% in Belgium, 0.5% in United States of America to 1.4% in Saudi Arabia (12-14). This may not reflect very accurate reporting though because it is not always easy to detect pregnancy in dialysis patients. Firstly, most of them are amenorrheic to begin with. Secondly, a borderline elevated serum ß hcg level may be found even in a non-pregnant dialysis patient. Nevertheless the above numbers give an idea about the general conception rate in the subset of women on dialysis.

Of the 318 pregnancies reported to NPDR (National Pregnancy in Dialysis Patients Registry) until their 1998 report, eight women had been pregnant three times while on dialysis and one woman even had 4 pregnancies while being on dialysis (12). Usually some residual renal function is present in the occasional pregnancy that reaches term in uremic women. From more than seven reports including 226 pregnancies in 196 women who became pregnant with a baseline serum creatinine level of 1.4 mg/ dl or greater, it is now known that their disease progresses more rapidly than disease in women with similar degrees of renal insufficiently who do not become pregnant (15-22).

The largest of these studies was a published by Jones and Hayslett in 1996 that included 82 pregnancies in 67 women with primary renal disease and a serum creatinine level of 1.4 mg/ dl or greater before conception. Overall, 43% of all women had a decline in glomerular filtration rate (GFR), which was defined as 25% or greater decline from baseline GFR. 8% recovered this decline within 6 months post-partum while another 10% suffered a new decline during this time period. The likelihood of an accelerated decline in renal function was greater in women with baseline serum creatinine greater than 2.0 mg/ dl. One of the 49 women with serum creatinine of 1.4-1.9 mg/ dl, 3 of the 9 women with serum creatinine of 2.0-2.4 mg/ dl and 4 of the 12 with serum creatinine above 2.5 mg/ dl experienced such an accelerated decline in GFR that they reached end-stage renal disease. 37% of all infants of the women in the above study had overt growth retardation. 59% compared to 10% in general population were premature and 59% of the women had to undergo a Caesarean – section (as compared to 20% in women with no renal disease).

Despite all these problems, overall infant survival was 93%. In sharp contrast, infant survival for women on dialysis was reported to be only 55% for those pregnancies reaching second trimester (13). 85% of their infants were premature. Three maternal deaths were reported to NPDR until 1998.

First et al. studied the effect of pregnancy on renal allograft function in a case control study at University of Cincinnati from 1967-1990. Twenty five pregnancies in 18 women were matched to long-term renal allograft survival seven years after pregnancy and 11.8 years after transplant to a group of well matched 26 female controls who had not been pregnant and 23 male control renal transplant recipients (23). Baseline serum creatinine was less than 2.0 mg/ dl in all but one of these women. They had 22 live births and 3 spontaneous abortions, 2 of the 3 abortions were in the same one woman whose creatinine clearance was 31-ml/ min and was advised against pregnancy. Renal allograft survival was similar between the three study groups at 11.8 years with no statistical difference. Thus, the authors concluded that pregnancy does not effect long-term allograft survival if mother's baseline serum creatinine is less than 2.0-mg/ dl.

There is a single controlled study that suggests graft function is adversely affected by pregnancy in which graft function of 22 women with 29 pregnancies was found to be 69% at 10 years compared to 100% for the control group of 38 female transplant recipients (24) This study has been criticized for the rarity of 100% graft function at 10 years in the control patients at any other transplant center. The bulk of the evidence suggests that graft function is usually not adversely affected by pregnancy if woman's baseline serum creatinine is less than 1.5-mg/ dl (15). General recommendations for advising pregnancy in women with renal transplants is baseline serum creatinine under 2.0 mg/ dl, good general health, easily controlled hypertension, proteinuria under 1 gm/ 24 hour and immunosuppression at maintenance levels.

Women's health issues in dialysis patients

Jung et al recently published a study stating that only eight of the forty eight hemodialysis patients interviewed reported being ever had hormone replacement therapy (HRT) (25). Over half had no pap smear and 38% of the women aged over 50 had no mammogram in the last two years.Holley et al found that only 5% of women over age 55 on dialysis were getting hormone replacement therapy while a contraindication to its use existed only in 4 % of women (6). Although 50% of the women under age 55 claimed to be sexually active, only 36% were using any form of birth control. Only 13% of the women stated that their nephrologist ever discussed birth control issues with them and another 19% reported that either a gynecologist or another primary care physician ever brought up this topic.

The overall risk of hip fracture in a woman aged less than 45 years on dialysis is about 76 times that of an age matched control woman from general population (26). If data from general population can be extrapolated to women with ESRD, hormone replacement therapy can reduce this risk of a major fracture in these women substantially. Cardiovascular disease is the leading cause of death in ESRD population. Again, looking at data from general non-ESRD population, hormone replacement therapy reduces this risk by upto 50%. A prospective randomized controlled trial showed that after 12 weeks of HRT in ESRD patients although triglycerides went up by 20% as expected, HDL also went up by 12%, LDL went down by 9% and most importantly LP(a) which has now emerged as an independent marker for cardiovascular disease went down by 36%. So far there is little if any other known therapy to bring LP(a) down to this extent. All the above parameters remained unchanged in control group (No HRT group). There was one vascular access thrombosis in HRT group and three episodes in control group. Hormone replacement therapy is grossly under prescribed in women with ESRD. According to one analysis of United States Renal Data System, only 10.8% of women on dialysis were getting HRT as compared to 34% in the general population (28). There is very little data on estrogen dosing in ESRD. One p harmacokinetic study of estrogen dosing suggests that estrogen dosing shall be halve din women with ESRD to achieve the same estradiol levels as control non-ESRD patient (29).

Summary

Menstrual abnormalities and reduced libido are very common in women with chronic renal failure. These disturbances usually persist even after replacement of renal function either by hemo or peritoneal dialysis. Furthermore, sexual dysfunction is very prevalent even in patients with well functioning renal transplants although it is still significantly less than from those on dialytic therapy. Physicians need to be more alert to these issues as patient may be shy to bring these up in discussion. Accelerated loss of renal function occurs with pregnancy if woman' s baseline serum creatinine is greater than 2.0-mg/ dl at the time of conception. This finding is helpful in more effective counseling of women with chronic renal failure who are contemplating to become pregnant. Maternal hypertension and increase in proteinuria seem to be t he major maternal morbidities during pregnancy. Many safe anti-hypertensive drugs are available to lower blood pressure in pregnancy. Of note is the information from two studies, one involving 46 infants and the other including 86 infants, showed no adverse effects of exposure to angiotensin converting enzyme inhibitors (ACE) in the first trimester (30). Women of childbearing age who may be receiving ACE inhibitors for their renoprotective effect need not discontinue them in planning for pregnancy if there is some reasonable assurance that pregnancy can be diagnosed promptly and the drug stopped at that point

Low birth weight and prematurity are common in infants born to mothers with chronic renal failure. Outcomes are improving with each passing decade. The bulk of the evidence suggests that pregnancy does not affect renal allograft function or survival if mother's serum creatinine is less than 1.5-2.0 mg/ dl. The major side effect in infants born to mothers taking cyclosporine is growth retardation with as many as 49% of them being growth retarded. Routine gynecologic cancer screening and hormone replacement therapy are not being done adequately in women on dialysis. One of the reasons for this may be that these women who are already coming three times a week to dialysis do not then go to a separate primary care physician who may take care of these issues. In this setting, it just seems appropriate that rather than forcing the patient to go to a primary care physician, the nephrologist shall assume this responsibility. Obviously, more manpower in nephrology is in turn needed to cope with all these demanding roles to provide the best possible patient care for women in dialysis.

References

1.	Procci WR, Goldstein DA, Adelstein J, Massry SG. Sexual dysfunction in the male patient with uremia: A reappraisal. Kidney Int 19;317-323, 1981.

2.	Toorians AW, Janssen E, Laan E, Gooren LJG, Giltay EJ, Oe PL, Donker AJM, Everaerd W. Chronic renal failure and sexual functioning: Clinical status versus objectively assessed sexual response. Nephrol Dial Transplant 12;2654-2663, 1997.

3.	Lim VS: Reproductive function in patients with renal insufficiency. Am J Kidney Dis 9; 363-367, 1987.

4.	Lim VS, Henriquez C, Sieverston G, Frohman IA: Ovarian function in chronic renal failure: Evidence suggesting hypothalamic anovulation. Ann Intern Med 93; 21-27, 1980.

5.	Gomez F, De La Cueva R, Wauters J-P, Lemarchand-Beraud T: Endocrine abnormalities in patients undergoing longterm hemodialysis: The role of prolactin. Am J Med 68; 522-530, 1980.

6.	Holley JL, Schmidt RJ, Bender FH, Francis D, Schiff M: Gynecologic and Reproductive issues in women on dialysis. Am J Kidney Dis 1997; 29:685-690.

7.	Zingraff J, Jungers P, Pelissier C, Nahoul K, Feinstein MC, Scholler R. Pituitary and ovarian dysfunction in women on hemodialysis. Nephron 1982; 30: 149.

8.	Ginsburg ES, Owen WF Jr: Reproductive endocrinology and pregnancy in women on hemodialysis. Semin Dial 1998; 6:105-116.

9.	Palmer BF. Sexual dysfunction in uremia. J Am Soc Nephrol 1999; 10: 1381.

10.	Swamy AP, Woolf PD,Cestero VM: Hypothalamic-pituitary – ovarian axis in uremic women. J Lab Clin Med 1979; 93: 1066.

11.	Diemont WL, Vruggink PA, Meuleman EJH, Doesburg WH, Lemmens WAJG, Berden JHM: Sexual dysfunction after renal replacement therapy. Am J Kidney Dis 2000; 35: 845.

12.	Souqiyyeh MZ Huraib SO, Saleh AGM, Aswad S: Pregnancy in chronic hemodialysis patients in the Kingdom of Saudi Arabia.: Am J Kidney Dis 1992; 19:235-238.

13. Okundaye IB, Abrinko P, Hou S: A registry for pregnancy in dialysis patients. Am J kidney Dis 1998; 31: 766-773.

14. Bagon JA, Vernaeuve H, De Muylder X Lafontaine JJ, Martens J, Van Roost G: Pregnancy and dialysis: Am J Kidney Dis 1998; 31: 756-765.

15. Hou S. Pregnancy in chronic renal insufficiency and end-stage renal disease: Am J Kidney Dis 1999; 33: 235-252.

16. Barcelo P, Lopez-Lillo J, Cabero L, Del Rio G: Successful pregnancy in primary glomerular disease: Kidney Int 1986; 30: 914-919.

17. Hou S, Grossman SD, Madias NE: Pregnancy in women with renal disease and moderate renal insufficiency: Am J Med 1985;78:185-194.

18. Imbasciatti E, Pardi G, Capetta P, Ambroso G, Bozzetti P, Pagliari B, Ponticelli C.: Pregnancy in women with chronic renal failure. Am J Nephrol 1986; 6: 193-198.

19. Cunningham FG, Cox SM, Handstand TW, Mason RA, Pritchard JA: Pregnancy in women with chronic renal failure. Am J Obstet Gynecol 1990; 163: 453-459.

20. Abe S: Pregnancy in glomerulonephritic patients with decreased renal function. Hypertens Pregnancy 1996; 15: 305-312.

21. Jungers P, Chauveau D, Choukroun G, Moynot A, Skhiri H, Houillier P, Forget D, Grunfeld JP: Pregnancy in women with impaired renal function. Clin Nephrol 19989;47:281-288.

22. Jones DC, Hayslett JP. Outcome of pregnancy in women with moderate or severe renal insufficiency. N Eng J Med 1996; 335: 226-232.

23. First MR, Combs CA, Weislttel P, Miodonovik M: Lack of effect of pregnancy on renal allograft survival or function. Transplantation 1995; 59: 472-476.

24. Salmela KT, Kyllonen LEJ, Holmberg C, Gronhagen-Riska C: Impaired renal function after pregnancy in renal transplant recipients. Transplantation 1993; 56: 1372-1375.

25. Jang C, Bell RJ, White VS, Lee PS, Dwyer KM, Kerr PG, Davis SR. Women's health issues in haemodialysis patients: Med J Aust 2001; 175: 292-3.

26. Stehman-Breen CO, Sherrard DJ, Alem AM, Gillen DL, Heckbert SR, Wong CS, Ball A, Weiss NS. Risk factors for hip fracture among patients with end-stage renal disease: Kidney Int 2000; 58:2000-2205.

27. Jung SP, Hae HJ, Won SY, Soon BK, Won KM, Hyun SC. Effects of hormonal replacement therapy on lipid and haemostatic factors in post-menopausal ESRD patients: Nephrol Dial Transpl 2000; 15: 1835-1840.

28. Stehman-Breen CO, Gillen D, Gipson D. Prescription of hormone replacement therapy in postmenopausal women with renal failure: Kidney Int 1999; 56: 2243-2247.

29. Ginsberg ES. Estrogen dosing in ESRD. J Clin Endocrinology and Metabolism 1996.

30. Briggs GG, Freeman RK, Yaffe SJ (eds): Drugs in pregnancy and lactation: Baltimore, MD. Williams and Wilkins, 1994.

Are Turf Battles and Managed Care To Blame For Late Referral of ESRD Patients

Onyekachi Ifudu

Introduction

In patients with chronic kidney disease, timely referral to a nephrologist increases the odds of identifying any treatable or reversible etiology [1-5]. Furthermore, prompt referral to the nephrologist permits early treatment of complications of kidney failure such as anemia, renal osteodystrophy and hypertension. In addition, preparation for renal replacement therapy requires sufficient time for patient education, modality selection, and access preparation.

Unfortunately, late referral to nephrologists of patients with chronic kidney disease is a major problem in the United States and is associated with increased morbidity, greater healthcare costs in the short-term and possibly increased mortality 6-10].

A key unresolved question in the causation of late referral of patients with chronic kidney disease, are the relative effects of managed care reforms (gate keeper effect) and primary care physician fear of losing their patients when they are referred to the nephrologist. This review will examine the epidemiology, other potential causes as well as consequences of late referral of patients with chronic kidney disease to the nephrologist.

Definition of "late referral"

An examination of the nephrology literature reveals a lack of consistency in how authors define or describe "late referral" to a nephrologist. A National Institute of Health consensus development panel on dialysis morbidity and mortality recommended that women with a serum creatinine concentration

≥ 1.5mg/dL (132.6 micromoles/ liter), and men with a serum creatinine concentration ≥ 2 mg/dL (176.8 micromoles/liter), should be referred to a nephrologist [1] for evaluation. However, several investigators have employed a higher threshold of serum creatinine to define late referral while many other shave defined late referral by time interval from referral to initiation of dialysis. These differences in the definition of late referral – use of residual renal function versus interval to renal replacement therapy have made it difficult to compare the outcomes of various studies.

Scope of the problem

Late referral to nephrologists of patients with chronic kidney disease is a major public health problem in the United States and is more pronounced in the inner-city [1-5]. Furthermore, it was quite prevalent even before the emergency of managed care "gate keeper" systems. A single-center study of 139 patients starting dialysis in Brooklyn in the early 1990s found that 57 percent of the patients did not receive prior nephrologic care [9]. In a report by Arora, et al.[4], 22 percent of new starts on dialysis had their first visit to a nephrologist less 4 months before initiation of dialysis. Another study of over 600 patient from six Boston area renal clinics found that the mean serum creatinine concentration at referral to the nephrologist was 3.2±1.6 mg/dL while theirmean glomerular filtration rate was 22.3± 8.91ml/min/ 1.73m^2 [11]. Confirming that late referral is not necessarily due to managed care bureaucracy or lack of insurance is a study of 220 patients with either Medicaid or medicare in Brooklyn whose serum creatinine concentration (mean± SEM) on referral was 3.5 ±0.21 mg/dL [7].

Late referral is however not limited to the US because a report from Europe reveals that 583 (26%) of 2236 new starts on dialysis were referred within one month before dialysis was needed [12].

Risk factors for delayed referral

Several studies have shown that, nonwhites (black and Hispanic patients) as well as older patients were at higher risk for late referral than their respective counterparts [6,7,10,13,14]. In a study of 220 medically-insured patients in Brooklyn it was found that late referral to the nephrologist (serum creatinine >4 mg/dL at referral) was six times more likely in nonwhites than whites with chronic renal failure (odds ratio 5.6; 95

CI, 1.52 to 20; $P = 0.008$)[7]. Also, late referral was more likely in patients over 55 years of age than in those 55 years or younger (odds ratio, 4.7; 95 CI, 1.37 to 16; $P = 0.01$)[7].

Our findings confirm and extend the results of surveys of primary care physicians and nephrologists that showed that delayed referral to the nephrologist was more prevalent in older than younger patients with chronic renal failure, and that dialysis was inappropriately being withheld in some older patients with chronic renal failure solely because of their age [13,14].

Causes of late referral

Though several causes (Table 1) have been postulated to explain late referral, none have been confirmed in a protocols study. Based on the prevalence of the problem prior to wide spread penetration of Managed care in the US market, it is unlikely that the managed care "gatekeeper" phenomenon is to blame [9]. Also, late referral of nonmanaged care patients with other types of health insurance would suggest a minimal role for managed care in this phenomenon [7].

It is postulated that there is a significant deficiency of knowledge among nonnephrologists about the unique nature of chronic kidney failure. The paucity of symptoms and signs in early chronic renal failure, and the fact that serum creatinine concentration becomes abnormal only after 60 to 70 percent of renal function is lost [15], predisposes to delayed recognition. The paucity of specific symptoms and signs in early renal insufficiency necessitates vigilance to detect renal failure. Depending on muscle mass, the serum creatinine concentration becomes elevated only after 60 to 70 percent of glomerular filtration rate is lost (Figure 1) [15].

In actuality, therefore, what is generally described as "early" or "mild" chronic renal failure, usually referring to a rise in serum creatinine concentration to 2 to 3 mg/dL represents a patient with less than 25 percent of normal glomerular filtration. The paucity of symptoms may also make patients less likely to seek nephrologic care until incipient uremia.

Consequences of late referral

Appropriate referral of a newly azotemic patient permits the nephrologist to: a) identify reversible or treatable causes of renal insufficiency; b) institute interventions to slow progression of renal failure, c) manage and/ or prevent complications of renal failure, and d) educate patients and their family about renal failure to select the best applicable renal replacement therapy (Table 2).

In patients with progressive renal disease, components of management include identification and treatment of reversible renal failure, adequate blood pressure control, proper nutritional support, good glycemic control and modulation of proteinuria in diabetic subjects, anemia correction with recombinant erythropoietin, and administration of vitamin D, phosphate binders, and calcium as treatment of early renal osteodystrophy to preempt severe secondary hyperparathyroidism.

In addition, as the need for renal replacement therapy approaches, discussion of options in uremia therapy is begun with patients' and the necessary psychosocial support provided to help them adjust to the stresses of uremia and its therapy. Finally, if maintenance hemodialysis is the chosen modality for renal replacement therapy, a vascular access to the circulation needs to be created before the need for dialysis arises. This comprehensive management is most appropriately provided by a nephrologist, enabling a timely and organized transition to renal replacement therapy.

When patients are referred late to the nephrologist, none of the above measures are able to be carried out by the clinicians. Consequently, muscle wasting, emesis and other uremic symptoms emerge in many such patients shortly after referral to the nephrologist, prompting initiation of dialysis without diagnostic evaluation or creation of a vascular or peritoneal access [4,5,9,16-21]. Intuitively late referral will result in poor outcomes and cannot under any circiunmstance be desirable. However, no randomized prospective studies show that appropriate referral to a nephrologist favorably effects either survival or cost of care in patients with progressive renal insufficiency. Several nonrandomized studies, however, conclude that early referral improves patient outcomes whereas delayed referral increases morbidity (acidosis and anemia), and prolongs hospital stay at initiation of dialysis [4,5,9,16-21].

Late referral lead to delayed initiation of dialysis, often via ineffecicient temporary hemodialysis catheters [7,9,16-18]. Astor, et al.[16], found that patients referred at least one month before initiation of dialysis were more likely than their counterparts to use an arteriovenous access at initiation of dialysis as well as six months later.

No where is the consequence of delayed refrerral more profound than in anemia management in PreESRD patients. Of 65,847 new starts on dialysisbin 1999 only 26.3 percent received prior treatement with erythropoietin [22]. Anemia worsens as kidney failure progresses and in fact the mean hematocrit of these new starts was 30.2 percent [22]. Aprreciating that anemia induces a spectrum of cardiovascular problems including left ventriculat hypertreophy, left ventricular dilatation as well as ischemic heart diseases, then the saliency of this issue is brought to the fore [23].

Left ventricular hypertrophy, an independent risk factor for mortality and cardiovascular disease accounts for about 50 percent of all deaths in ESRD [22]. It is widely recognized that this excess mortality in dialysis patients is attributed in part to risks during progressive renal insufficiency [23]. However, there are conflicting reports with regards to the effect of late referral or timing of initiation of dialysis on mortality in dialysis patients [19-21,24-31].

Late referral and survival on dialysis

While several studies have found that late referral to a nephrologist shortens survival in dialysis patients [21,26-31], others have found no relation between timing of referral and subsequent death risk (19,20,24,25].

Roubicek, et al. [19], reported equivalent 3,12 and 60 month survival in 97 patients referred less than 16 weeks before initiation of dialysis and the other 173 referred earlier. Similarly, Schmidt, et al. [20], found that referral within 30 days of needing dialysis had no significant effect on survival. In a prospective 39 month single center study in Brooklyn, neither serum creatinine concentration nor albumin at initiation of dialysis had an effect on survival [24]. Confirming these reports is a study published in 2001 showing no statistically significant difference in 3 year survival between early and late starts [25].

However, other investigators have shown that late referral shortens survival [26-31] and PreESRD erythropoietin use confers a surviival benefit in the first 19 months of ESRD [21]. In fact, Jungers, et al. [30], found longer 5 year survival if preESRD nephrologic care was greater than 6 months, and Bonomini, et al. [31], observed higher 12 year survival (85% vs 51%) in patients who started dialysis earely (creatinine clearance >10 mL/min) than in patients who started late (creatinine clearance <4 mL/min).

What is the explanation for the conflicting findings about late referral and survival. Possibilities include the fact that there indeed may not be a significant relation between them or that some of the studies had design flaws. Also, it is possible that it is difficult to determine the cut-off point to define late referral [32]. If uremia-indued injury is universally present in most patients that are being studied, an arbitrarily selected cutoff point to define late referral may not yeild a difference between the two groups. Furthermore, because of the morbidity and other significant bad effects associated with late referral, a randomized study to examine the effect on survival will be impractical and unethical.

Combating Late Referral

Corrective measures to combat delayed referral of patients with chronic renal failure may be more likely to be successful if targeted at subgroups of patients at higher risk than others. Combating delayed referral of patients with chronic renal failure will entail collaborative efforts by primary care physicians and nephrologists, since primary care physicians usually treat most patients with hypertension and diabetes mellitus, the two most common causes of chronic renal failure [22].

An aggressive public education campaign (similar to cholesterol education campaign) emphasizing that early in kidney failure that there is a lack of symptoms bu that such patients should obtain nephrologic care can be directed at patients who have diseases known to cause kidney failure. Education of healthcare providers as trainees will emphasize vigilance as a necessary tool to pick up chronic kidney disease early in it's cause.

Onyekachi Ifudu, MD, MSc
Renal Disease Division
Department of Medicine
SUNY Downstate Medical Center
Brooklyn, New York

References

1. Morbidity and Mortality of Renal Dialysis: An NIH Consensus Conference Statement. Consensus Development Conference Panel. Ann Intern Med 1994;121:62-70.
2. Striker G. Report on a workshop to develop management recommendations for the prevention of progression in chronic renal failure. J Am Soc Nephrol 1995;5:1537-1540.
3. Eadington DW. Delayed referral for dialysis: higher morbidity and higher costs. Seminars in Dialysis 1995;8:258-260.
4. Arora P, Obrador GT, Ruthazer R, et al. Prevalence, predictors, and consequences of late nephrologic referral at a tertiary care center. J Am Soc Nephrol 1999;10:1281-6.
5. Levin A. Consequences of late referral on patient outcomes. Nephrol Dial Transplant 2000;15:S8-13.
6. Bloembergen WE, Young EW, Woods JD, et al. Factors associated with late referral among new dialysis patients in the US [Abstract]. J Am Soc Nephrol. 1997;8:A0870.
7. Ifudi O, Dawood M, Iofel Y, Valcourt JS, Friedman EA. Delayed referral of black, Hispanic, and older patients with chronic renal failure. Am J Kidney Dis 1999;33:728-733.
8. Obrador GT, Ruthazer R, Arora P, Kausz AT, et al. Prevalence of and factors associated with suboptimal care before initiation of dialysis in the United States. J Am Soc Nephrol 1999;10:1791-800.
9. Ifudi O, Dawood M, Homel P, Friedman EA. Excess morbidity in patients starting uremia therapy without prior care by a nephrologist. Am J Kidney Dis 1996;28:841-845.
10. Winkelmayer WC, Glynn RJ, Levin R, et al. Determinants of delayed nephrologist referral in patients with chronic kidney disease. Am J Kidney Dis 2001;38:1178-84.
11. Kausz AT, Khan SS, Abichandani R, et al. Management of patients with chronic renal insufficiency in the Northeastern United States. J Am Soc Nephrol. 2001;12:1501-7.
12. Lameire N, Van Biesen W. The pattern of referral of patients with

end-stage renal disease to thenephrologist—a European survey. Nephrol Dial Transplant 1999;14 (Suppl 6):16-23.

13. Mendelssohn DC, Kua TB, Singer P. Referral for dialysis in Ontario. Arch Intern Med 1995;155:2473-2478.

14. Sekkarie MA, Moss AH. Withholding dialysis on ESRD patients by nephrologists and primary care physicians [Abstract]. J Am Soc Nephrol 1996;7:1463.

15. Levey AS, Madaio MP, Perrone RD: Laboratory assessment of Renal Disease: Clearance, Urinalysis and Renal Biopsy. *In* Brenner BM, Rector FC, The Kidney eds (4th), 1991, W.B. Saunders Company, Philadelphia, PA, pp919-968.

16. Astor BC, Eustace JA, Powe NR, et al. Timing of nephrologist referral and arteriovenous access use: the CHOICE Study. Am J Kidney Dis 2001;38:494-501.

17. Goransson LG, Bergrem H. Consequences of late referral of patients with end-stage renal disease. J Intern Med 2001;250:154-9.

18. Holland DC, Lam M. Suboptimal dialysis initiation in a retrospective cohort of predialysis patients—predictors of in-hospital dialysis initiation, catheter insertion and one-year mortality. Scand J Urol Nephrol 2000;34:3411-7.

19. Roubicek C, Brunet P, Huiart L, et al. Timing of nephrology referral: influence on mortality and morbidity. Am J Kidney Dis 2000;36:35-41.

20. Schmidt RJ, Domico JR, Sorkin MI, et al. Early referral and its impact on emergent first dialyses, health care costs, and outcome.Am J Kidney Dis 1998;32:278-83.

21. Finkn J, Blahut S, Reddy M, et al. Use of erythropoietin before the initiation of dialysis and its impact on mortality. Am J Kidney Dis 2001;37:378-55.

22. United States Renal Data Systems. USRDS. 2001 Annual Data Report. National Institutes of Health, National Institutes of Diabetes and Digestive and Kidney Diseases; Bethesda, MD, 2001.

23. Levin A. Prevalence of cardiovascular damage in early renal disease.Nephrol Dial Transplant 2001;16 Suppl 2:7-11.

24. Ifudu O, Dawood M, Homel P, et al. Timing of initiation of uremia therapy and survival in patients with progressive renal disease. Am J Nephrol 1998;18:193-8.

25. Korevaar JC, Jansen MA, Dekker FW, et al. When to initiate dialysis: effect of proposed US guidelines on survival.Lancet 2001;358:1046-50.

26. Sesso R, Belasco AG. Late diagnosis of chronic renal failure and mortality on maintenance dialysis. Nephrol Dial Transplant 1996;11:2417-20.

27. Innes A, Rowe PA, Burden RP, et al. Early deaths on renal replacement therapy: the need for early nephrological referral. Nephrol Dial transplant 1992;7:467-71.

28. Chandna SM, Schulz J, Lawrence C, et al. Is there a rationale for rationing chronic dialysis? A hospital based cohort study of factors affecting survival and mordibity.BMJ 1999;18:217-23.

29. Stoves J, Bartlett CN, Newstead CG. Specialist follow up of patients before end stage renal failure and its relationship to survival on dialysis. Postgrad Med J 2001;77:586-8.

30. Jungers P, Massy ZA, Nguyen-Khoa T, et al. Longer duration of prediaysis nephrological care is associated with improved long-term survival of dialysis patients. Nephrol Dial Transplant 2001;16:2357-64.

31. Bonomini V, Feletti C, Scolari MP, Stefoni S. Benefits of early initiation of dialysis. Kidney Inter 1985;28:S57-S59.

32. Ifudu O. Timing of initiation of uremia therapy: where is the science? Int J Artif Org 1997;20:601-602.

Table 2

Consequences of Late Referral

1. Missed opportunity to identify reversible or treatable causes of chronic kidney disease
2. Excess morbidity associated with complications of renal failure – anemia, hypertension, cardiovascular disease, etc
3. Lack of adequate preparation for renal replacement therapy and exploration of options in uremia therapy
4. Possible increased cost of care
5. Delayed initiation of renal replacement therapy
6. Increased mortality among those with end-stage renal disease on dialysis
7. Unmeasured effects, i.e., starting uremia therapy under emergency conditions without adequate preparation is a turn-off. May foster a negative attitude about dialysis therapy and may result in noncompliance

Figure 1

Relation between serum creatinine concentration and glomerular filtration rate

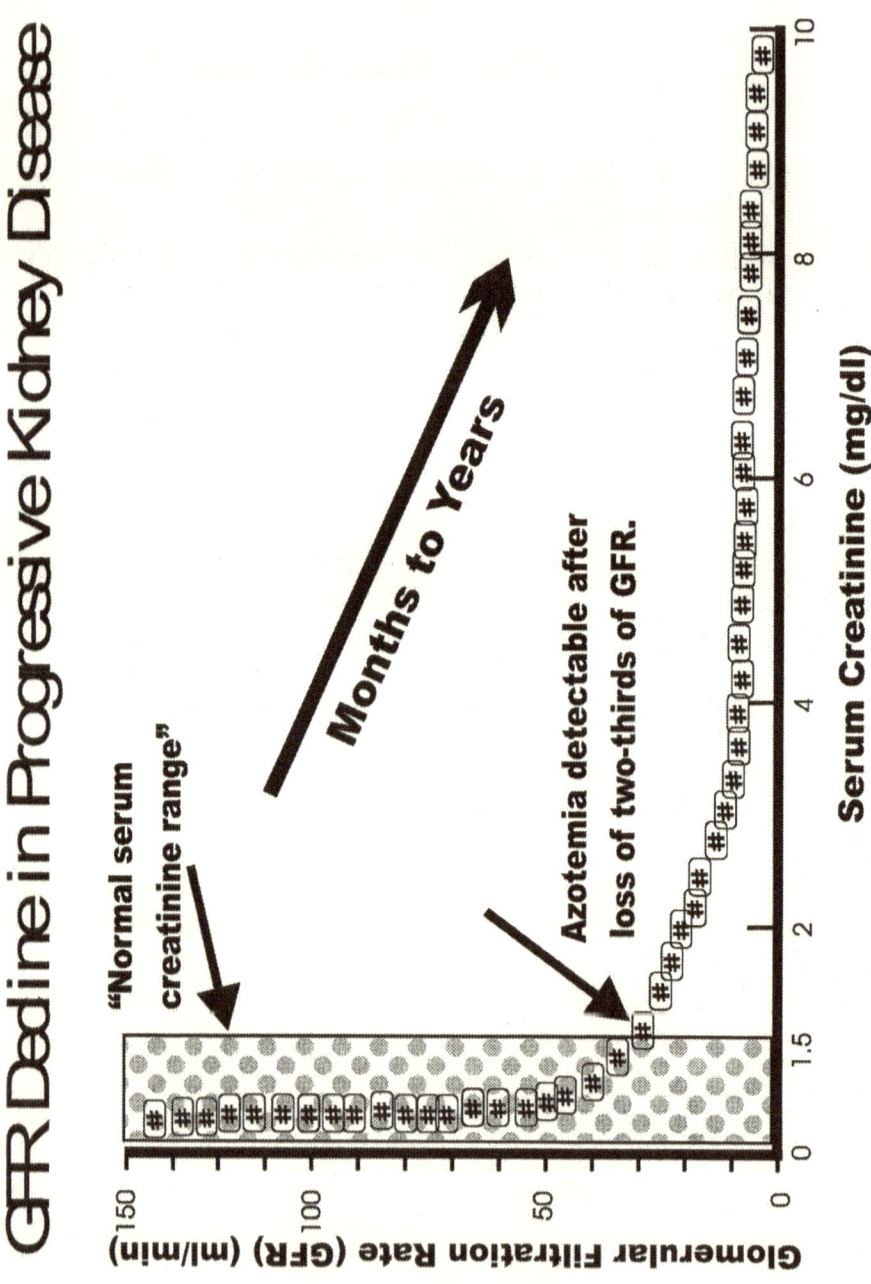

Emergency Room Care of ESRD Patients: What Nonnephrologists Need To Know

Yalem Woredekal, M.D.

Introduction

The number of patients with end-stage renal disease has been increasing steadily for the last two decades in the USA and other developed countries. USRDS for 2001 reports 360,000 US patients were receiving renal replacement therapy at the end of 2000 [1]. Diabetes is the leading cause of ESRD, and during 2000, 44.5% of newly diagnosed ESRD patients were diabetics, with this rapid increase mostly seen in people above the age of 65. Although the mortality rate of dialysis patients has been improving steadily compared to other patients, it is still high, with the two commonest causes of death cardiovascular disease and infection.

As the number of ESRD patients increase, the number of visits to the emergency room by ESRD patients has also increased, and Emergency Department physicians are increasingly presented with the challenge of handling acute problems in the dialysis population. Although dialysis treatment in an emergency room is given in consultation with the nephrologist, only a knowledgeable physician who is aware of the special problems of dialysis patients can give effective emergency care.

Common presentations of ESRD patients to an Emergency Room

The pathophysiology of end-stage renal disease predisposes patients to a number of unique medical conditions. Fluid and electrolyte imbalance, infection, and problems related to vascular access commonly bring them to an emergency room, but there are few studies that have looked into the pattern of such dialysis patient visits. Gruss et al prospectively examined

83 outpatient hemodialysis patients to find common emergency room diagnoses and identify the possible risk factors associated with patients who were frequently seen in an ER [2].

Fifty-five of the 83 patients (66%) had 118 emergency room visits in 1998; 51% of these visits were initiated by the patients themselves. The four most frequent diagnoses were infection 19.5% (23/118), trauma 15.3% (18/118), gastrointestinal symptoms 15.3% (18/118), and problems related to vascular access 12% (14/118). 30% (36/118) of emergency consultations needed hospital admission, and infectious disease processes accounted for the highest percentage of these. The risk factors for repeated visits (more than 3 times) were: age (68.9 vs. 61.4), lower hematocrit (31.6 vs. 34.4%), and lower Kt/V (0.99 vs. 1.1).

In another prospective study, Sacchetti et al looked at 100 dialysis patients presenting initially to an emergency room for acute care in one tertiary care facility over a 3 month period [3]. Of the 100 patients, 80 were on hemodialysis and 20 on peritoneal dialysis. Forty-six patients discharged from the emergency room while the remaining 54 patients were either admitted to the hospital or transferred to the dialysis unit. The common presenting symptoms were: shortness of breath, chest pain, abdominal pain, and weakness. Those patients (19/54) who required interventional dialysis in the emergency room had shortness of breath as their presenting symptom.

Management of acute medical problems in ESRD patients

Congestive heart failure (CHF): Shortness of breath secondary to congestive heart failure is the most common cause of emergency room visits for anuric ESRD patients. Interdialytic fluid gain and acutely accelerated hypertension are the two commonest cause of CHF and, ultimately, dialysis is needed to remove this excess fluid. However, even in hospitals with active dialysis units, it may take several hours to initiate dialysis when the unit is closed. Given the respiratory distress involved, initial stabilization is the responsibility of emergency room physicians, and pharmacologic agents can be used effectively for management of congestive heart failure in dialysis patients until dialytic therapy is available.

Depending upon the severity of the presenting symptoms, different techniques can be utilized to treat acute congestive heart failure in these patients. Supplemental oxygen can be administered either through a mask, nasal prongs or, in severe cases, endotracheal intubation. Pharmacologic agents used to treat acute CHF are aimed at maximizing left ventricular function through cardiac preload and afterload reduction. Sublingual nitroglycerin (NTG) (0.4 to 0.8mg), or transdermal nitroglycerin (1/2 to 2 in of paste) can be uses for preload reduction. Oral captopril, nifedipine, or intravenous nitroprusside have been found to be effective for afterload reduction [5, 6]. Morphine sulfate has a vasodilator action, and can also be used to treat acute CHF. Because of its respiratory depressant effects, morphine should be used with caution in this group of patients.

In a retrospective study phlebotomy was shown to be an effective acute treatment for CHF in dialysis patients [7]. This technique should be used only those patients with a reasonable hematocrit level (>30%).

Hyperkalemia: Serious hyperkalemia is common in ESRD patients, seen in about 10% [8], and accounts for considerable morbidity and mortality. In one study it was reported that hyperkalemia was the reason for emergency dialysis 24% of the time [4]. It is one of the more common acute life-threatening metabolic emergencies seen in any emergency room. Early diagnosis and empiric treatment of hyperkalemia is dependent in many cases on the emergency room physician's ability to recognize the electrocardiographic (EKG) manifestations of hyperkalemia. The classic EKG manifestations of hyperkalemia include peaked T waves, prolongation of PR interval, loss of P wave, widening of the QRS complex (sine wave), ventricular fibrillation, and asystole [9,10]. These changes may be influenced by factors such as extracellular fluid pH, calcium and sodium concentrations [9], and the rate of increase in serum potassium [10].

Although a serum potassium above 6.5 mmol/L is usually associated with some of the above described EKG changes, it has been reported that no corresponding EKG changes may be seen in some patients with extremely high potassium levels of more than 9.0 mmol/L [11]. Besides the cardiac effect, hyperkalemia may also result in paresthesia and muscle weakness, progressing to a flaccid paralysis that typically spares the diaphragm. Deep tendon reflexes are depressed or absent. Cranial nerves are rarely involved and sensory changes are minimal [12].

As the treatment for hyperkalemiais is safe as long as it is done properly, and delay in treatment can result in unpredictable death, it is wise to have a low threshold for initiation of emergency treatment. Although dialysis is the definitive treatment for hyperkalemia in ESRD patients, dialysis treatment may be delay by a number of hours because of logistic reasons; other non-dialytic measures should be instituted to treat hyperkalemia in these patients.

Non-dialytic treatment for hyperkalemia

Direct Membrane Antagonism: Calcium directly antagonizes the effect of hyperkalemia on the myocardium without lowering the serum potassium level. Calcium in injection form is available as gluconate or chloride salt. The recommended dose is 10 ml of 10% of calcium gluconate or chloride intravenously over 10 minutes. The onset of action is less than 3 minutes. The EKG should be continuously monitored and the dose can be repeated in 5 minutes if there is no improvement in the EKG or if it deteriorates after initial improvement. The duration of action is 30-60 minutes. There are case reports of sudden death in patients receiving intravenous calcium while also receiving digitalis [13]. For this reason IV calcium should be given with caution.

Redistribution of Potassium into Cells: Insulin stimulates cellular potassium uptake independent of its effect on cellular glucose uptake [14]; its action is dose dependent. The recommended dose is 10 units of regular insulin as a bolus along with an intravenous bolus of 25-50 grams of dextrose as a 50% solution. This dose of insulin can lower the serum potassium by 1 mmol/L. The onset of action is less than 20 minutes and the maximum effect is seen in 30 to 60 minutes [14]. Dextrose solution should be avoided in patients with a high serum glucose level (>250mg/dl), and concomitant hyperkalemia- they can be treated with insulin alone.

Albuterol : It has been shown that administration of the selective β_2 adrenoreceptor agonist (albuterol) by intravenous infusion (0.5 mg over 15 minutes) to patients with renal failure will lower serum potassium by 1 mmol/L in 30 to 60 minutes [14,15]. Similar effect has also been shown with the use of nebulized albuterol in high dose. Serum potassium declines by 0.6mmol/L after inhalation of 10 mg of albuterol, and by about 1 mmol/L with 20 mg. The onset of action is 30 minutes and the duration 2-4 hours. Mild tachycardia is the most common side effect reported with the use of high dose albuterol. The hypokalemic effect of albuterol may not be seen by in patients taking nonselective beta-adrenoreceptor blockers. It has been observed among ESRD patients not taking beta-blockers that as many as 40% are resistant to the hypokalemic effect of albuterol [16]. The mechanism for this resistance is not well understood, but, for this reason, albuterol treatment should not be considered as the only treatment for urgent hyperkalemia in ESRD patients.

Elimination of Potassium from the Body: Sodium polystyrene sulfonate (SPS Kayexalate) is a resin that exchanges sodium for potassium in the gastrointestinal tract, there by allowing potassium elimination from the body. Each gram of resin binds approximately 0.6 mmol of potassium in vivo [16], although the effect is highly variable and unpredictable. It can be given orally or by retention enema. The rate of potassium removal is relatively slow, requiring approximately 2 to 4 hours for full effect. There are many case reports of patients who have developed intestinal necrosis after exposure to SPS in sorbitol as an enema or as an oral agent [17,18].

Infections in ESRD Patients

Infection is the second leading cause of death in ESRD patients [1]. When annual pulmonary infectious mortality rate in ESRD patients was compared to the general population, the mortality was 14-16 fold higher in dialysis patients, and approximately two fold higher in renal transplant patients [19].

Infections in hemodialysis patients

Vascular access infections are a major source of morbidity and mortality among hemodialysis patients, and accounts for up to 10% of all deaths, and approximately three-fourths of all deaths caused by infection. 16-25% of all hospital admissions are secondary to vascular access related infection [20].

The incidence of vascular access related infection is highest with the use of a central venous catheter, followed by arteriovenous grafts. Silent infection in old nonfunctional clotted prosthetic A-V grafts has recently been recognized as a frequent cause of bacteremia among hemodialysis patients [20]. High proportions of infections related to the vascular access are caused by staphylococcus organisms, which carry high rates of recurrence, metastatic complications, and morality.

Hemodialysis patients with vascular access related infection may present with fever and/or pain around the catheter or graft site, or even with spontaneous bleeding from the graft. Bleeding from an access can be due to rupture of the graft, and is usually secondary to infection. It can be a life- threatening emergency. Once bleeding is controlled by applying pressure, a surgeon should be contacted to either ligate or remove the graft. Since the cause is most often due to infection, it is appropriate to administer IV antibiotics before the surgery. Therefore it is crucial for an emergency room physician to identify this emergent condition and take appropriate measures. The treatment for vascular access infections without bleeding is IV antibiotics and, in most cases patients should be admitted to hospital.

Infections in CAPD Patients

Acute peritonitis is the most common cause of infection in patients on continuous peritoneal dialysis (CAPD). Organisms causing peritonitis in these patients are gram-positive in 65-75%, gram- negative in 25-30%, and other organisms in less than 5% of cases. The diagnosis of peritonitis in CAPD patients is usually made by observing cloudy dialysate outflow, with increased leukocyte counts (>100 cells/ml) predominantly polymorphonuclear cells. Abdominal pain and other symptoms, although often present, may be absent in the early stage of infection.

The initial treatment of acute peritonitis includes first a quick dialysate exchange to lavage the peritoneum and remove some bacteria, followed by administration of antimicrobial agents either intraperitoneal or intravenously. The choice of antibiotics depends upon the gram stain result if available, otherwise the current recommendation for empiric antibiotic treatment for PD related peritonitis is to use a combination of first generation cephalosporin and caftazidime [21]. This combination therapy has a good coverage against both gram-positive and gram-negative organisms. Both can be mixed in the same dialysate bag and can be administered as an initial treatment. Emergency room physicians should be able to provide the initial management of peritonitis.

Infections in kidney transplant patients

The risk of infection, particularly opportunistic infections in renal transplant patients is high specially during the initial post transplant period when they are highly imunosuppressed. In recent years, as organ transplantation has become more successful and a greater percentage of patients are being rehabilitated and returned to the general community;

transplant recipients are also affected by typical infection like the general population.

The major immunosuppressive drugs (cyclosporin and tacrolimus) are metabolized utilizing the hepatic cytochrome P_{450} linked enzyme, thus interacting with drugs that use the same enzyme for their metabolism. For example antimicrobial agents like naficilline, rifampin, and isonizide up-regular cyclosporin metabolism resulting in lower blood level of cyclosporin causing acute rejection. On the other hand macrolides (erythromycin > clarithromycin > azthromycin) and antifungal agents (ketaconazole > fluconazole) down-regulate cyclosporin metabolism causing high blood level of cyclosporin, increasing the risk of cyclosporin toxicity. The challenge for emergency room physicians is to be aware of the potential interaction between immunosuppressive drugs and antimicrobial agents.

Yalem Woredekal, M.D.
Renal Disease Division
Department of Medicine
SUNY Downstate Medical Center
Brooklyn, New York

References

1. United States Renal Data System (USRD) 2001 Annual Data Report. The National Institute of Health, National Institute of Diabetes, Digestive and Kidney Disease, Bethesda, MD 2001.
2. Gruss E, Carmelo C, Fernandes C, et al. Why do ambulatory hemodialysis patients go to emergency service. Nefrologia 2000;20(4):336-341.
3. Sacchetti A, Harris RL, Patel K, Attewell R. Emergency Department Presentation of Renal Dialysis Patients: Indications for EMS Transport directly to dialysis centers. J Emerg Med 1991;9:141-144.
4. Sacchetti A, Stuccio N, Panebianco P, Torres M. ED Hemodialysis for treatment of Renal Failure Emergencies. Am J Emerg Med 1999;17(3):305-307.
5. Angeli P, Chiese M, Caregaro L, et al. Comparison of sublingual captopril and nifedipine in immediate treatment of hypertension emergencies. Arch Intern Med 1991;151:678-682.
6. Sacchetti A, McCabe J, Torrres M, Harris RL. ED Management of acute congestive heart failure in renal dialysis patients. Am J Emerg Med 1993;11(6):644-647.
7. Eiser AR, Lieber JJ, Neff MS. Phlebotomy for pulmonary edema in dialysis patients. Clinic Nephrol 1997;47(1):47-49.
8. Tzamaloukas AH, AvasthiPS. Temporal profile of serum potassium concentration in non-diabetic and diabetic outpatients in chronic dialysis. Am J Nephrol1987;7:101-109.
9. Fisch C. Relation of electrolyte disturbances to cardiac arrhythmias. Circulation 1973;47:408-419.
10. Surawicz B. Relationship between electrocardiogram and electrolytes. Am Heart J 1967;73:814-834.
11. Szerlip HM, Weiss J, Singer J. Profound hyperkalemia without electrocardiographic manifestation. Am J Kidney Dis 1986;7:461-465.
12. Weiner M, Epsein FM. Signs and symptoms of electrolyte disorders.

Yale J Biol Med 1970;43:76-109.

13. Shrager MW. Digitalis intoxication. A review and report of forty cases with emphasis on etiology. Arch Inter Med 1957;100:881-893.

14. Allon M, Copkney C. Albuterol and insulin for treatment of hyperkalemia in hemodialysis patients. Kidney Int 1990;38:869-872.

15. Lens SM, Montoliu J, Cases A, Campistol JM, Revert L. Treatment of hyperkalemia in renal failure Nephrol Dial 1Transplant 1989;4:228-232.

16. Allon M, Dunlay R, Copkney C. Nebulized albutrol for acute hyperkalemia in patients on hemodialysis. Ann Intern Med 1989;110:426-429.

17. Wooten FT, Rhodes DF, Lee WM, Fitts CT, Colonic necrosis with Kayexalate-sorbitol enemas after renal transplantation. Ann Intern Med 1989;111:947-949.

18. Gerstman BB, Kirkman R, Platt R. Intestinal necrosis associated with postoperative orally administered sodium polystyrene sulfonate in sorbitol. Am J Kidney Dis 1992;20:159-163.

19. Sarnak MJ, Jaber BL. Pulmonary infectious mortality among patients with end-stage renal disease. Chest 2001;120(6):1883-1887.

20. Ayus JC, Sheikh-Hamad D. Silent infection in clotted hemodialysis access graft. J Am Soc Nephrol 1999;9:1314-1317.

21. Keane WF, Bailie GR, Boeschoten E et al. Adult Peritoneal Dialysis-Related Peritonitis Treatment Recommendations 2000 UPDATE. Perit Dial Int 2000:20:396-411.

Preventing Infections in Hemodialysis Patients: Are We Doing Enough?

Anthony J. Joseph, MD

Introduction

Infections cause excess morbidity and mortality in hemodialysis patients. Although dialysis centers strive to prevent infections among their patients, they often fail this objective. Reasons underlying this lack of success are multifactorial. Firstly, patients on hemodialysis remain immunosuppressed by persistent uremia, and, consequently, are more susceptible to infections. In uremia, polymorphonuclear leucocyte (PMNLs), responsible for defense against bacterial infection, are dysfunctional because of undesirable effects of iron overload, increased intracellular calcium, uremic toxins, bio-incompatible dialyzer membranes, and accelerated apoptosis. Hemodialysis patients also exhibit significant alterations of T- and B-cell function including suboptimal reactions to vaccines.

Secondly, h emodialysis procedure and dialysis unit structure afford all the necessary elements for successful propagation of infections. Vascular accesses are cannulated and used for several hours in a milieu where immunocompromised patients are exposed to contaminated devices and people via the hands of healthcare workers. Hemodialysis units constitute large reservoirs of blood-borne viruses and bacterial microorganisms.

Thirdly, nephrologists and dialysis staff members are not sufficiently proactive in their battle protocols to preempt infections. Implementation and adherence to a comprehensive infection control program is subadequate. Violations to sound infection control practices are frequent indialysis units. The Centers for Disease Control and Prevention (CDC) reports that, in 2000, 73% of centers lacked a dedicated ddrug preparation room, only 58% tested patients for anti-HCV antibody, and no more than 57.7% of patients received at least 3 doses of hepatitis B vaccine. Concurrently, the number of central venous catheters used for dialysis has doubled from 1995 to 2000. Obviously, infection prevention should be a priority for each center.

Scope of the problem

Infection is the second leading cause of death in both diabetic and nondiabetic patients with end-stage renal disease (ESRD) [1]. Mailloux et al. reported that infections were responsible for 36% of all deaths occurring at North Shore University Hospital over a 16-year period [2]. Among prevalent hemodialysis patients between 1997 and 1999, the 2001 annual report of the United States Renal Data System (USRDS) indicated that infections accounted for 19.9% of all deaths in the 20-40 year age group, 16% and 13.7% of deaths in the 45-64 and 65 year and older age groups, respectively [1]. The USRDS might even underestimate death rates due to infectious causes in patients receiving hemodialysis because of coding errors in ESRD death notification forms. For instance, in a recent report by Joseph and Lundin, an infectious illness was the actual cause of death in 25% of cases thought to be due to cardiac arrest of unknown cause [3].

The 2001 USRDS also reported that septicemia accounted for 62% of the infection category in the 20-44 year age group and 81% in the 45 year and older age group [2]. Further to the point, Sarnak and Jaber, using data from the National Center for Health Statistics and the USRDS, found aht mortality secondary to sepsis was 100 to 300-fold higher in ESRD patients on dialysis when compared with the general population [4]. Most dialysis centers strive to prevent infections among their patients, but it is not uncommon to fail this objective. This review analyzes the causes of this failure.

Why do infections occur more often in hemodialysis patients?

Causes of an increased infection rate in hemodialysis patients are multifactorial. Firstly, dialysis patients are immunosuppressed and, consequently, are more susceptible to infections [5-7]. Secondly, hemodialysis units constitute an ideal milieu for the transmission of infections [8]. Finally, as this report will substantiate, nephrologists and dialysis staff members are ineffective in minimizing infectious complications.

Why are hemodialysis patients immunocompromised?

Uremia, particularly if associated with malnutrition, modulates profoundly the immune system [6,8]. Polymorphonuclear leucocytes (PMNLs) are the main cell defense against bacterial linfections. PMNLs dispose of bacteria by a sequence of efficiently coordinated events consisting of adhesion to vascular endothelial at the site of infection, ingestion and killing of bacteria through the generation of reactive oxygen species and release of enzymes [9]. Impairment of the host defense, due to altered PMNL functions, is primarily responsible for this susceptibility to infections displayed by ESRD patients [6]. In uremic people, PMNL dysfunction may be generated by iron overload, increased intracellular calcium, uremic toxins, bio-incompatible dialyzer membranes, and accelerated apoptosis.

Before the introduction of recombinant human erythropoietin (rHuEPO), several reports established a connection between iron overload due to frequent blood transfusions and an increased rate of infection [10,11]. In vitro studies found that iron suppressed phagocytosis. For example, PMNLs from healthy controls incubated with iron manifest inhibition of phagocytosis [12,13]. Conversely, treatment with erythropoietin decreases serum ferritin levels and improves phagocytosis [14]. The adverse effects of iron on the phagocytic function of PMNLs may be explained by direct action of iron on cell membrane or by generation of reactive oxygen species capable of damaging PMNLs [13,15].

The validity of early clinical studies implicating iron overload as an independent risk factor for infection is disputed on the basis of inappropriate patient selection or faulty analysis [16]. For example, two reports included patients recently treated for infection or dialyzed through central venous catheters [17,18]. It is speculated that infections raised serum ferritin levels, as opposed to

iron overload having been responsible for an increased risk of infection. In a recent report by Patruta and colleagues, the legitimacy of high ferritin level as a cause of PMNL dysfunction in hemodialysis patients with low transferring saturation (TSAT) was addressed by measuring the functional capacity of PMNLs from 3 groups of hemodialysis patients sorted by ferritin levels [19]. Leucocyte function was not affected in people with serum ferritin levels lower than 60 :g/L. Oppositely, PMNLs from hemodialysis patients with serum ferritin values between 100 :g/L and 350 :g/L showed mild impediment of phagocytosis but profound inhibition of intracellular killing of bacteria as well as significant reduction of oxidative burst. The third patient group, with ferritin levels greater than 650 :g/L and TSAT inferior to 20% had still a greater impairiment of PMNL functions. Chronic inflammation or infection was not the cause of hyperferrinemia in this study since 21 out of 26 patients had plasma levels of C-reactive protein (CRP) lower than the detection limit (<0.5 mg/dL). One patient had a CRP value within the normal range (<1.0 mg/dL) and four showed slightly elevated CRP values (1.18 to 3.0 mg/dL). One of these patients belonged to group I, one to group II, and two to group III [19].

Caution is warranted about overtreatment of hemodialysis patients with intravenous iron, but a safe level of serum ferritin in those subjects remains to be determined. After reviewing the world literature on iron overload and risk of infection, the Anemia Work Group of the National Kidney Foundation-Kidney Disease Outcomes Quality Initiative (NKF-KDOQI) inferred that maintaining a serum ferritin below 800 ng/mL is unlikely to expose patients with chronic kidney disease to an increased risk of bacterial infections [20].

Clinical observations suggest that parathyroid hormone (PTH) affects leucocyte function [21]. Chronic and excessive PTH activity increases basal levels of PMNL cytosolic calcium ($[Ca^{2+}]$), reduces calcium signal after activation of Fc(RIII receptor, and impairs phagocyosis in people with renal failure [21]. Calcium channel blockers disrupt the effect of PTH on PMNLs and improve their phagocytosis in humans [21].

All PMNL functions are also inhibited by uremic toxins which accumulate in the serum of ESRD patients as a result of reduced excretion or increased synthesis during dialysis. Several toxins including granulocyte inhibitory proteins, degranulation inhibiting proteins, immunoglobulin light chains, and chemotaxis inhibiting proteins have been isolated from patients on hemodialysis and chronic ambulatory peritoneal dialysis [6].

Hemodialysis with a cuprophane membrane may be associated with adverse reactions including neutropenia, leukocyte dysfunction, and mild pulmonary hypertension due to neutrophil migration to the lungs [22]. Several studies conclude that those complications are generated by complement activation via the alternative pathway following contact of neutrophils with bio-incompatible membranes such as cuprophane [22,23]. The intensity of complement activation decreases with biocompatible or less complement activating membranes such as polysulfone and polyacrionitrile. Cuprophane dialyzers suppress phagocytic function during dialysis [22]. Contrastingly, this abnormality does not occur with biocompatible membranes. Vanholder et al. found that, during the first 3 months after initiating hemodialysis, the glycolytic response and reactive oxygen production were substantially lower in patients dialyzed with cuprophane when compared with those treated with polysulfone membranes (24, 25].

To the contrary, Rosenkranz and colleagues reported that the production of reactive oxygen species was higher with cuprophane as opposed to polysulfone membranes [26]. Data on the production of reactive oxygen species in subjects dialyzed with cuprophane are conflicting [9].

Another plausible explanation for host defense impairment is the down modulation of L-selectins and upregulation of granulocyte adhesion receptor Mac-1 (CD11b/CD18 or CR3) when bio-incompatible membranes are used for hemodialysis [27]. Selectins are responsible for the initial rolling interaction of leukocytes with the vascular endothelium and Mac-1 assures firm adhesion of leucocytes to endothealial cells [28,29]. Low selectin and high Mac-1 expression on granulocytes leading to a decreased ratio between L-selectin and Mac-1 could impair the host defense against infections in hemodialysis patients [30].

Out of all leucocytes, PMNLs have the shortest half-life;[31] they rapidly die in vitro by apoptosis [32]. In vivo, mature circulating PMNLs spend about 12 hours in the bloodstream, and subsequently migrate into normal tissues or are attracted to inflamed tissues, where they undergo apoptosis and are engulfed by tissue phagocytes. Leucocytes harvested from ESRD patients and cells from healthy volunteers exposed to uremic plasma undergo accelerated apoptosis [33]. In addition, the dysfunctional pattern of normal PMNLs undergoing apoptosis is similar to that of uremic PMNLs which demonstrate altered oxidative responses, and impaired chemotaxis, aggregation, and phagocytosis [34]. Jaber et al. have speculated that "uremia-induced" apoptosis may be partly responsible for the {MNL dysfunction commonly observed in uremic patients [35]. According to a recent report by Rosenkranz and colleagues, both biocompatible and bio-incompatible dialyzer membrance scould also accelerate apoptosis in human PMNLs [36].

Patients on h emodialysis exhibit significant alterations of B- and T-cell function [37]. The predominant reduction of Tl-cell function in uremia can be tested by decreased cutaneous responsiveness to several antigens [38].

By contrast, global parameters of B-cell function do not show relevant differences between dialysis patients and healthy controls [38,39]. Neither the amount

of total immunoglobulins nor the IgG subclasses in serum are reduced. Examples of T- and B-cell dysfunction have been well documented in subjects with renal failure. For instance, ESRD patients infected with hepatitis B have a relatively acute course of infection and do not eradicate this virus as healthy subjects do. This leads to a chronic carrier state (30% of infected ESRD patients as opposed to 5% in the normal population) [40,41].

There is also diminished seroconversion after vaccination with influenza, tetanus, or diphtheria [42- 44]. The mechanisms leading to B and T cell dysfunction are indirect. The intrinsic function of both types of cell is intact when they are provided with normal signaling from antigen-presenting cells (APCs) [37, 45]. Uremia has a profound effect on APCs which, subsequently, inhibits B and T cell activation [37, 45]. Girndt, analyzing the molecular aspects of T- and B-cell function in uremia, proposes that two major components of immune deviation are relevant. Firstly, impaired expression of the costimulatory molecule B7-2 (CD86) on monocytes causes reduced signaling which leads to low activation of helper T cells [37]. This dysfunction is associated with uremia and may be improved by high-efficiency renal replacement therapy [46]. The other component is inflammatory activation of APCs mainly due to dialyzer membranes [37].

Dialysis unit: an ideal milieu for transmission of infections

Hemodialylsis procedure and dialysis unit structure assemble all the necessary elements for a successful propagation of dangerous infections. Hemodialysis process requires the use of vascular access which is a suitable portal of entry. Vascular accesses, cannulated and used for several hours, are implicated in up to 50% to 73% of all bacteremias in hemodialysis patients [47, 48]. Additionally, many susceptible and immunocompromised hosts receive their treatment simultaneously in a milieu where contaminated devices, equipment, environment surfaces as well as infected patients or hosts constitute large reservoirs of blood-borne viruses and bacterial microorganisms [49,50].

Usually, hemodialysis patients are infected by certain blood-borne viruses such as Hepatitis B Virus (HBV), Hepatitis C Virus (HCV), and Human Immunodeficiency Virus (HIV). In 2000, the prevalence of HBV, HCV, HIV among hemodialysis patieints was respectively 0.9, 8.4, and 1.5% [49]. Both HBV and HCV are transmitted by percutneous or permucosal exposure to infectious blood or body fluids [51]. Although chronic HBV and HCV carriers are key to the transmission of those viruses, hepatitis B antigen has been also found on environmental surfaces [52]. The route of HCV transmission in unknown in approximately 10% of cases [53]. Several publications reveal that most HBV and HCV outbreaks among dialysis patients occur by cross-contamination due to poor infection control practices [53-56]. Thus far, HIV transmission has not been reported in U.S. dialysis centers, but it has occurred in other countries, as a result of reusing syringes or access needles [57, 58].

As many as 50% to 62% of hemodialysis patients are carriers of Staphylococcus Aureus [50]. In hemodialysis centers, the reported prevalence of vancomycin resistant enterococcus (VRE) in stool samples ranges from 1% to 9% [59]. Hemodialysis patients are also colonized with methicillin-resistant coagulase negative Staphylococcus (CNS), methicillin-resistant Staph aureus (MRSA), and multidrug-resistant gram rods including strains of Pseudomonas aeruginosa, Acinetobacter species [51].

Bacterial infections follow invasion of pathogens present in or on patients or contamination of dialysis fluids and equipment [60]. Endogenous bacteria first colonize the skin and/or nares and later cause clinical infection [60]. Generally, colonization is due to the propagation of pathogens from a colonized or infected patient to a host via the hands of negligent health-care workers [51, 60].

Exogenous pathogens caused several outbreaks which resulted from substandard dialyzer reprocessing technique, inadequate treatment of municipal water, or faulty machine design [61-63]. In a report of an epidemic of pyrogenic reactions and gram-negataive bacteremia occurring in a hemodialysis center, Jackson et al. indicated that bacterial and endotoxin concentrations of water used to prepare dialysate and reprocess hemodialyzers exceeded allowable concentrations recommended by the Association for the Advancement of Medical Instrumentation [61]. Dialysis tubing and connector left submerged in flush containers during priming were responsible for an epidemic of gram negative bacteremia in a Canadian unit [62]. Three clusters of gram-negative bloodstream infections at hemodialysis centers in Canada, the United States, and Israel resulted from contamination of the waste-handling option (WHO), a drain port designed to dispose of saline used to flush dialyzers [63].

Bacteremia has been also linked to exogenous drug contamination. Grohslopf et al. reported ten cases of serratia liquefaciens septicemia from contamination of Epoietin Alfa at a hemodialysis center [64]. There were 21 episodes of heparin-infusion related bacteremia in an Australian unit [65].

Renal community is not doing enough to prevent infections among hemodialysis patients

Preventing transmission of bloodborne viruses and pathogenic bacteria among dialysis patients necessitates implementation of a comprehensive infection control program [51]. The Centers for Disease Control and Prevention (CDC) recommends that components of such a program include infection control practices specifically designed for hemodialysis centers, routine serologic testing and immunization, surveillance, training and education [51].

Infection control practices for hemodialysis units include the following: [51], 1) Staff members should wear gloves whenever caring for patients or touching dialysis equipment; 2) Hands should be washed after gloves are removed and between patient contacts, as well as after touching blood, body fluids, secretions, or contaminated items; 3) Antiseptic hand rub can be employed instead of water washing if hands are not visibly soiled; 4) Objects taken to a dialysis station could be contaminated and should be disposed of or cleaned and disinfected before being returned to a common clean area; 5) Unused medications or supplies taken to a patient's station should not be returned to a common clean area or used on other patients; 6) Each unit should have written protocols for cleaning and disinfecting surfaces and equipments.

Implementation and adherence to such a program are frequently lacking. Major violations to infection control practices are regularly observed in hemodialysis units. For example, staff members lift up the cover of a waste disposal container with or without gloves and subsequently touch patients, equipment, use a telephone and type on a keyboard. At times, health care workers have to be reminded of hand washing after they remove their gloves. It seems that they forget that latex or vinyl gloves can be associated with leaks and contamination [65]. In seeking for suitable areas to cannulate a dialysis access, staff members, not wearing sterile gloves, may palpate the puncture site which was already cleaned and disinfected. Certain hospitals utilize common supply carts which are wheeled back and forth from the acute dialysis center to intensive care units. This practice increases the chance of cart contamination with multidrug-resistant organisms.

An additional measure to defeat infection in a dialysis facility is to prepare medications in a designated room or area. Medications should be delivered separately to each patient. The CDC, in their 2000 annual report on the National Surveillance on Dialysis-Associated Diseases in the United States, showed that the incidence of HbsAg was lower when medications were ddrawn up in a dedicated room as opposed to the dialysis station (0.05% vs 0.13%, P<0.05) [49]. Similarly, the incidence of anti-HCV was lower when medications were prepared in separate room instead of a medication quarter within the dialysis treatment area (0.19% vs 0.30%, P<0.05) [49]. Unfortunately, only 21% of surveyed centers employed a designated room for drug preparation [49].

Routinely, all patients should be tested for HBV and HCV infection. Referring dialysis centers should communicate HBV test results to receiving hospitals when infected patients are being admitted [56]. Although the vaccination rate has increased from 1983 to 2000, only 57.7% of patients received at least 3 doses of hepatitis B vaccine in the United States [49]. The prevalence of anti-HBs antibody, whose presence indicates immunity to HBV infection, was only 37.6% [49]. According to the CDC, only 58% of surveyed centers in 2000 tested their patients for anti-HCV antibody whose prevalence was 8.4% at those centers. During the same year, dialyzers were reused in 80% of those polled hemodiallysis centers [49]. One can infer that several units where reuse was practiced did not test their patients for anti-HCV antibody. Since the prevalence of anti-HCV was higher in centers which reused dialyzers on anti-HCV positive patients (8.7%) as opposed to those which did not (7.6%) PP=0.004)[49], it is possible that outbreaksk of hepatitis C may go unnoticed in those centers if absence of anti-HCV testing persists.

Over the past 24 years, dialysis centers in the U.S. have successfully decreased the prevalence of HBV infection from 7.8% to 0.9% [49]. The CDC recommends hepatitis B vaccination for all susceptible chronic hemodialysis patients and staff members [51,66]. Pre-ESRD and home hemodialysis patients should also be vaccinated since they may require in-hospital dialysis. After the last vaccine dose, all vaccines should be tested for antibody to hepatitis B surface antigen (anti-HBs). Health-care workers and patients who do not convert should be re-vaccinated with three additional doses and retested for response [51].

To its list of recommendations [51], the CDC fails to add reduction of dialysis catheter use as a mean to prevent infections. As noted above, vascular accesses were implicated in up to 50% to 73% of all bacteremias in hemodialysis patients. The incidence of infection caused by vascular access is highest when it is a central venous catheter and lowest when it is a native arteriovenous fistula. In its 2000 report on the National Surveillance of Dialysis-Associated Diseases (NSDAD) in the U.S., the CDC found that the rate of access-related bacteremias per 200 patient-

month was 0.25 for fistulae, 0.53 for grafts, 4.84 for cuffed catheters, and 8.73 for non-cuffed catheters [49]. Of particular concern is that more patients from surveyed centers received dialysis through catheters, 19,471 in 1995 versus 67,511 in 2000 [49].

Because of its long half-life, vancomycin is frequently administered to hemodialysis patients. Consequently, ESRD patients have played a significant role in the growing problem of vancomycin resistance [67]. In three reports, 12% to 22% of hospitalized patients infected or colonized with vancomycin resistant enterococcus (VRE) were receiving hemodialysis [67]. Further to the point, a study analyzing data from 49 hospitals found aht hemodialysis and peritoneal dialysis were independent risk factors for VRE bacteremia [68]. Over a 5-year period (1995-2000), the number of centers reporting VRE infected patients grew from 12% to 32% [49]. Additionally, three of the first five subjects identified with vancomycin-intermediate staphylococcus aureus (VISA) or glycopeptide – intermediate staphylococcus aureus (GISA) were on chronic hemodialysis [69].

It is clear that antibiotics, particularly vancomycin, must be judiciously used to prevent epidemics of antimicrobial-resistant pathogens. Data from the NSDAD indicated 93% of centers

reported employing at least one measure to encourage appropriate antimicrobial use [49]. The reason for antibiotherapy was recorded by 63% of centers. A written policy on antimicrobial use and an automatic stop order were adopted respectively in 36% and 31% of centers. Approval for certain antibiotics was needed in 22% of units which participated in this national survey.

There are data suggesting that cefazolin, a first-generation cephalosporin, could be a safe alternative to vancomycin [70]. It is important to note that cefazolin blood levels were therapeutic 48-72 hours after dosing [70]. Tokars, speaking for the Hospital Infections Program (CDC), indicates the role of postdialysis defazolin is clearest for continuing therapy in ESRD patients when the isolated organism is susceptible to first-generation cephalosporins [67]. Cefazolin also may be used for empiric therapy when the risk of MRSA is small, infection does not appear to be life threatening, or vascular access is unlikely the source of infection [67].

In summary, infection imposes a major burden on hemodialysis patients. Although preventing infections among hemodialysis patients is challenging, this objective should be a priority for every center. All staff members, from medical directors to housekeepers, as well as patients must be trained and re-trained about good infection control behaviors and techniques. Primary care physicians and nephrologists should make a concerted effort to minimize the use of central venous catheters in new or established hemodialysis patients. Nephrologists anticipate that an anti-staphylococcal vaccine, providing minimal and temporary protection, may be perfected soon [71].

References

1.	United Renal Data System, USRDS 2001 Annual Data Report: Atlas of End-Stage Renal Disease in the United States, National Institute of Health, National Institute of Diabetes and Kidney Diabetes and Kidney Diseases, Bethesda, MD, 2001
2.	Mailloux LU, Belluci AG, Wilkes BM et al. Mortality in dialysis patients: Analysis of the causes of death. Am J Kidney Dis 1991; 18:326-35.
3.	Joseph AJ, Lundin AP. Coding errors in ESRD death notification forms (HCFA-2746) falsely increase cardiac death rate. J Am Soc Nephrol 1999, 10:286A
4.	Sarnak MJ, Jaber BL. Mortality caused by sepsis in patients with end-stage renal disease compared with the general population. Kidney Int 2000; 58:1758-64.
5.	Descamps-Latscha B, Herbelin A, Nguyen AT. Immune system in Uremia. Seminars in Nephrology 1994; 14:253-60.
6.	Hörl WH. Neutrophil function and infections in uremia. Am J Kidney Dis 1999; 33:ppxiv-xlviii.
7.	Cohen G, Haag-Weber M, Hörl WH. Immune dysfunction in uremia. Kidney Int 1997; 52:S70-S82.
8.	Haag-Weber M, Dumann H, Hörl WH. Effect of malnutrition and uremia on impaired cellular host defence. Miner Electrolyte Metab 1992; 18:174-85.
9.	Ward RA. Phagocytic cell function as an index of biocompatibility. Nephrol Dial Transplant 1994; 9 (Suppl 2):46-56.
10.	Tielemans CL, Lenclud CM, Wens R, et al. Critical role of iron overload in the increased susceptibility of haemodialysis patients to bacterial infections. Beneficial effects of desferrioxamine. Nephrol Dial Transplant 1989;4:883-7.

11.	Cantinieaux B, Boelaert J, Hariga C, et al. Impaired neutrophil defense against Yersinia enterolitica in patients with iron overload who are undergoing dialysis. J Lab Clin Med 1988; 111:524-8.
12.	van Asbeck BS, Marx JJM, Struyvenberg A et al. Effect of iron (III) in the presences of various ligands on the phagocytic and metabolic activity of human polymorphonuclear leucocytes. J Immunol 1984; 132:85106.
13.	Hoepelman IM, Jaarsma EY, Verhoef J et al. Polynuclear iron complexes impair the function of polymorphonuclear granulocytes. Br J Haematol 1988;68:385-9.
14.	Boelaert JR, Caninieaux BF, Hariga CF, et al. Recombinat erythropoietin reverses polymophonuclear granulocyte dysfunction in iron-overload dialysis patients. Nephrol Dial Transplant 1990;5:504-17.
15.	Hoepelman IM, Jaarsma EY, Verhoef J et al. Effect of iron on polymorphonuclear granulocyte phagocytic capacity: rolle of oxidation state and effect of ascorbic acid. Br J Haematol 1988;70:495-500.
16.	Eschbach JW, Adamson JW. Iron overload in renal failure patients: Changes since the introduction of erythropoietin therapy. Kidney Int 1999;55 (Suppl. 69):S35-S43.
17.	Seirfert A, Von Herrath D, Schaefer K. Iron overload, but not treatment with desferrioxamine favors the development of septicemia in patients on maintenance hemodialysis. Q J Med 1987, 65:1015-24.
18.	Hoen B, Kessler M, Hestin D, et al. Risk factors for bacterial infections in haemodialysis adult patients: A multicenter prospective survey. Nephrol Dial Transplant, 1990;5:130-4.
19.	Patruta SI, Edlinger R, Sunder-Plassman G, et al. Neutrophil impairment associated with iron therapy in hemodialysis patients with functional iron deficiency. J Am Soc Nephrol 1998;9:655-653.

20.	NKF-K/DOQI Clinical Practice Guidelines for Anemia of Chronic Renal Failure. New York, NY, National Kidney Foundation, 2001.
21.	Massry SG, Smogorzewski M. Dysfunction of polymorphonuclear leucocytes in uremia: Role of parathyroid hormone. Kidney Int 2001;59 (Suppl 78): S195-S196.
22.	Craddock PR, Fehr J, Dalmasso AP, et al. Hemodialysis leukopenia: Pulmonary vascular leukostasis resulting from complement activation by dialyzer cellophane membrane. J Clin Invest 1977;59:870-88.
23.	Craddock PR, Fehr J, Brigham KL et al. Complement and leukocyte-mediated pulmonary dysfunction in hemodialysis. N Engl J Med 1977;296:769-74.
24.	Vanholder R, Ringoir S, Dohndt A et al. Phagocytes in uremic and hemodialysis patients: A prospective and cross sectional study. Kidney Int 1991;39:320-27.
25.	Vanholder R, Ringoir S. Polymorphonuclear cell function and infection in dialysis. Kidney Int 1992;42:S91-S95.
26.	Rosenkranz AR, Templ E, Traindl O et al. Reactive oxygen product formation by human neutrophils as an early marker for biocompatibility of dialysis membranes. Clin Exp Immunol 1994;98:300-05.
27.	Himmelfarb J, Zaoui P, Hakim RM. Modultion of granulocyte LAM-1 and Mac-1 during dialysis: A prospective, randomized controlled trial. Kidney Int 1992;41:388-398.
28.	Lawrence MB, Springer TA. Leukocytes roll on a selectin at physiologic flow rates: distinction from and prerequisite for adhesion through integrins. Cell 1991;31:859-873.
29.	Springer TA. Adhesion receptors of the immune system. Nature 1990;346:425-34.

30.   Thylén P, Fernvik E, Haegerstrand A, Lundahl J, et al. Dialysis-induced serum factors inhibit adherence of monocytes and granulocytes to adult human endothelial cells. Am J Kidney Dis 1997;29:78-85.

31.   Sendo F, Tsuchida H, Takeda Y, et al. Regulation of neutrophil apoptosis: Its biological significance in inflammation and the immune response. Hum Cell 1996;9:215-222.

32.   Squier MKT, Sehnert AJ, Cohen JJ. Apoptosis in leucocytes. J Leukoc Biol 1995;57:2-10.

33.   Cendoroglo M, Jaber BL, Balakrishnan VS, et al. Neutrophil apoptosis and dysfunction in uremia. J Am Soc Nephrol 1999;10: 93-100.

34.   Whyte MK, Meagher LC, Macdermot J et al. Impairment of function in aging neutrophihls is associated with apoptosis. J Immunol 1993;33:45-48.

35.   Jaber BL, Cendoroglo M, Balakrishnan VS et al. Apoptosis of leucocytes: Basic concepts and implications in uremia. Kidney Int 2001;59:S197-S205.

36.   Rosenkranz AR, Peherstorfer E, Körmöczi GF, et al. Complement-dependent acceleration of apoptosis in neutrophils by dialyzer membranes. Kidney Int 2001;59:S216-S220.

37.   Girndt M, Sester M, Sester U, et al. Molecular aspects of T- and B-cell function in uremia. Kidney Int 2001;59:S206-S211.

38.   Sester U, Girndt M, Kaul H, et al. Immunodeficiency with advanced renal failure: Altered regulation of B7-1 and B-7 expression. J Am Soc Nephrol 1997;8:76.

39.   Okasha K, Saxena A, el Bedowey MM, et al. Immunoglobulin G subclasses and susceptibility to allosensitization in humans. Clin Nephrol 1997;48:165-72.

40.   Crosnier J, Jungers P, Courouce AM, et al. Rnadomised placebo-controlled trial of hepatitis B surface antigen vaccine in French hemodialysis units: II, Haemodialysis patients. Lancet 1981;1: 797-800.

41.   Benhamou E, Courouce AM, Jungers P, et al. Hepatitis B vaccine: Randomized trial of immunogenicity in hemodialysis patients. Clin Nephrol 1984:21:143-147.

42.   Rautenberg H, Proppe D, Schütte A, et al. Influenza subtype-specific immunoglobulin A and G responses after booster versus one double-dose vaccination in hemodialysis patients. Eur J Clin Microbiol Infect Dis 1989;8:897-900.

43.   Girndt M, Pietsch M, Köhler H. Tetanus immunization and its association to hepatitis B vaccination in patients with chronic renal failure. Am J Kidney Dis 1995;26:454-60.

44.   Kreft B, Klouche M, Kreft R, et al. Low efficiency of active immunization against diphtheria in chronic hemodialysis patients. Kidney Int 1997;52:212-16.

45.   Girndt M, Köhler H, Schiedhelm-Weick E, et al. T-cell activation defect in hemodialysis patients: Evidence for a role of the B7/CD28 pathway. Kidney Int 1993;44:359-365.

46.   Kaul H, Girndt M, Sester M et al. Initiation of hemodialysis treatment leads to T cell activation in patients with end stage renal disease. Am J Kidney Dis 2000;35-611-616.

47.   Kessler M, Hoen B, Mayeux D, et al. Bacteremia in patients on chronic hemodialysis. A multicenter prospective survey. Nephron 1993;64:95-100.

48.   Quarles LD, Rutsky EA, Rostand SG. Staphylococcus aureus bacteremia in patients on chronic hemodialysis. Am J Kidney Dis 1985;6:412-19.

49.   Tokars JI, Frank F, Alter MJ, et al. National surveillance of dialysis-associated diseases in the United States, 2000.

50.   Centers for Disease Control and Prevention. Guideline for intravascular device-related infections. Am J Infect Control 1996;24:262-93.

51.   Centers for Disease Control and Prevention. Recommendations for preventing transmission among chronic hemodialysis patients. MMWR Morb Mortal Wkly Rep 1002;50(RR05):1-43.

52.	Bond WW, Favero MS, Petersen NJ, et al. Survival of hepatitis B virus after drying and storage for one week. Lancet 1981;1:550-51.

53.	Centers for Disease Control and Prevention. Recommendations for prevention and control of Hepatitis C Virus (HCV) infection and HCV-related chronic disease. MMWR Morb Mortal Wkly Rep 1998;47(RR19):1-39.

54.	Syndman DR, Bryan JA, London WT, et al. Transmission of hepatitis B associated with hemodialysis: role of malfunction (blood leaks) in dialysis machines. J Infect Dis 1976;134:562-70.

55.	Syndman DR, Bryan JA, Macon EJ, et al. Hemodialysis-associated hepatitis: report of an epidemic with further evidence on mechanisms of transmission. Am J Epidemiol 1976;104:563-70.

56.	Hutin YJ, Goldstein ST, Varma JK, et al. An outbreak of hospital-acquired hepatitis B virus infection qmong patients receiving chronic hemodialysis. Infect Control Hosp Epidemiol 1999;20:731-35.

57.	Velandia M, Fridkin SK, Cardenas, Cardenas V, et al. Transmission of HIV in dialysis center. Lancet 1995;345:1417-22.

58.	El Sayed NM, Gomatos PJ, Beck-Sague CM et al. Epidemic of human immunodeficiency virus in renal dialysis centers in Egypt. J Infect Dis 2000;181:91-97.

59.	Tokars JI, Gerh T, Parrish J et al. Vancomycin-resistant enterococci colonization at selected outpatient hemodialysis centers [Abstract]. Infect Control Hosp Epidemiol 2000;21:101.

60.	Jarvis WR. The epidemiology of colonization. Infect Control Hosp Epidemiol 1996;17:47-52.

61.	Jackson BM, Beck-Sague CM, Bland LA, et al. Outbreak of pyrogenic reactions and gram-negative bacteremia in a hemodialysis center. Am J Nephrol 1994;14:85-59.

62.	Humar A, Oxley C, Sample ML, et al. Elimination of an outbreak of gram-negative bacteremia in a hemodialysis unit.

63. Centers for Disease Controla nd Prevention. Outbreaks of gram-negative bacterial bloodstream infections traced to probable contamination of hemodialysis machines. Canada, 1995, United States, 1997; and Israel, 1997. MMWR Morb Mortal Wkly Rep 1998;47:55-58.

64. Grohskopf LA, Roth VR, Feikin DR, et al. Serratia liquefaciens from contamination of Epoietin Alfa at a hemodialysis center. N Engl J Med 2001;344:1491-97.

65. Playford EG, Looke DF, Whitby M, et al. Endermic nosocomial gram-negative bacteraemias resulting from contamination of intravenous heparin infusions. J Hosp Infect 1999;42:21-26.

66. CDC. Immunization of health-care workers: recommendations of the Advisory Committee on Immunization Practices (ACIP) and the Hospital Infection Control Practices Advisory Committee (HICPAC). MMWR 1997;46(RR-18):1-42.

67. Tokars JI. Vancomycin use and antimicrobial resistance in hemodialysis centers. Am J Kidney Dis 1998;32:521-23.

68. Edmond MB, Wallace SE, Pfaller MA et al. Surveillance at 49 US medical centers for VRE bacteremia. 34th Annual Meeting of the Infectious Disease Society of America, New Orleans, LA, 1996 (abstr 49).

69. CDC. Staphylococcus aureus with reduced susceptibility to vancomycin—Illinois, 1999.MMWR Morb Mortal Wkly Rep 1999;48:1165-67.

70. Fogel MA, Nussbaum PB, Feintzeig ID, et al. Cefazolin in chronic hemodialysis patients: A safe, effective alternative to vancomycin. Am J Kidney Dis 1998;32:401-409.

71. Shinefield H, Black S, Fattom A, et al. Use of a Staphylococcus aureus conjugate vaccine in patients receiving hemodialysis. N Engl J Med 2002;346:491-496.

Optimizing Anemia Management in Chronic Kidney Disease

Robert Provenzano, M.D.

Introduction

Anemia of chronic kidney disease (CKD) inevitably occurs when renal function deteriorates to less than 30% of normal. Prior to the availability of recombinant human erythropoietin (rHuEPO), the anemia in CKD patients was accepted as a relatively asymptomatic manifestation of progressive renal deterioration and was treated with packed red blood cell transfusions only in the most extreme symptomatic cases [1-15].

Since the availability of rHuEPO our understanding of the clinical significance of anemia has opened a new are of study. In 1997 the National Kidney Foundation Dialysis Outcomes Quality Initiative (NKF-DOQI) published their review of the anemia in chronic kidney disease and established evidence based guidelines for its management [a]. This review will focus on the increasing prevalence of CKD in addition to anemia screening, supplementation of iron and defining optimal dosing of rHuEPO.

Scope of the Problem

Estimates of the number of US population with CKD may run as high as 6,200,000 as defined by a serum creatinine greater than 1.5 mg/dL [b]. As the majority of this population are under the care of general practitioners, internal medicine specialists, and family practitioners, recognition of anemia as a co-morbid condition is of paramount importance. Historically anemia in CKD has been given little attention by physicians.[c-5]. Current data has shown that the mortality, hospitalization rate and cost of patient care (per member per month) increases as hematocrit decreases [d]. Anemia in CKD is typically normochromic, normocytic and asymptomatic [6]. Indeed, due to the chronicity of the anemia, most patients are able to tolerate very low hemoglobins. This "asymptomatic state" is misleading as studies evaluating the correction of anemia have shown that patient quality of life, role functioning and energy levels improve significantly [e]. The cardiovascular consequences of anemia are severe and include progressive left ventricular hypertrophy, exacerbation of angina and a precipitating factor for congestive heart failure. Other adverse consequences of anemia include reductions in aerobic capacity and cognition.

Evaluation and screening of anemia

The National Kidney Foundation's K-KOQI clinical practice guidelines recommend that patients with serum creatinines greater than 2.0 mg/dL be screened for anemia [15]. Men and postmenopausal women with hemoglobins less than 12 g/dL and premenopausal women with hemoglobins less than 11 g/dL should be evaluated to determine the cause for their anemia.

Iron deficiency contributes to 30% of anemia in this population [7] and should be excluded by first screening serum iron, total iron binding capacity and serum ferritin levels. If iron deficiency is identified, iron replacement, as will be defined later, should be initiated and reevalulation for correction of anemia be made. Based on the practitioner's evaluation of the patient's nutritional status, consideration for folate or B12 deficiency should also be made and measurements of these vitamins ordered if appropriate. Barring this, if serum iron levels are normal, initiation of treatment with rHuEPO is recommended. Appropriate dosing should result in a prompt correction o fhte anemia. If the anemia does not respon despite the proper dosage of rHuEPO and adequate serum iron levels, consideration of a hematologic workup with bone marrow biopsy to assess the status of erythroid precursors should be made. This is an uncommon occurrence and rarely should hematologic evaluation be required. (Figure 1)

Recombinant human erythropoieetin therapy

Endogenous erythropoietin is a 30.4 kDa glycoprotein secreted primarily by the kidney and to a smaller and insignificant amount by the liver. It is immunologically and biologically indistinguishable from recombinant erythropoietin. Recombinant human erythropoietin was approved by the Food and Drug Administration for treatment of renal anemia in 1989. Erythropoietin binds to receptors on erythroid burst-forming units (BFU) and colony forming unit (CFU) in the bone marrow leading to increase erythropoiesis.

Although there are few specific principles on the dosing of rHuEPO, the response to recombinant rHuEPO is dose dependent and has been traditionally dosed three times weekly in hemodialysis patients [1,6]. Initial doses on hemodialysis range from 50 to 200 U/kg three times per week IV. Data is available that shows subcutaneous administration to be more cost advantageous as the drug dose is decreased taking advantage of the improved pharmacokinetics of this route of administration. Recent work Owen, et al [10] and Provenzano et al [11] have shown that weekly doses of recombinant rHuEPO, SQ, as initial therapy in CKD patients can maintain hemoglobins in a target range. Indeed unpublished communications suggest that less frequent dosing ranging from every other week to every four weeks may also maintain target hemoglobins in this population.

Dosing behavior for the CKD population has been extrapolated from experience gained in the hemodialysis population. Once target hemoglobins are reached consideration for decrease in the frequency in the dose should be made to improve patient compliance and ease of administration. Often this requires an increasing dose with decreasing frequency of administration. Periodic monitoring of iron stores should be made monthly at first and following stabilization of rHuEPO doses on a quarterly basis.

Iron therapy

Iron deficiency remains the most common cause for resistance to recombinant rHuEPO therapy [7]. THe accelerated rate of erythropoiesis increases iron requirements typically beyond the ability of oral iron administration to compensate [17]. MacDougall et al [12] has shown that the number of rHuEPO dose adjustments decreases when comparing patients who receive no iron therapy, oral iron therapy and IV iron therapy. There are many reasons oral iron may be an inadequate method in replenishing iron store sin CKD patients. Oral iron has a low intestinal absorption rate even in h ealthy persons [17]. Additionally patient compliance may be poor because of GI upset. Physiologically the regulation of intestinal iron transport dramatically impairs iron absorption at transferring saturations above 15-20%, that level recommended for optimal erythropoiesis [12].

[12] In view of this information parenteral iron supplementation should be considered to reverse negative iron balance in CKD patients.

Initial concerns that IV iron posed serious infection risks in dialysis patients resulted in some timidity in using this route of administration. Several well-designed prospective cohort studies though have failed to show relationship between the rates of serious infection and either body iron stores or IV iron dose [13]. Several IV iron products (iron dextran, iron gluconate, and iron sucrose) are available with varying advantages and disadvantages as well as dosing recommendations. The clinician's goals should be maintenance of serum ferritin levels greater than 100 ng/mL and transferring saturations greater than 20%. There are additional measurements useful in assessing iron status including reticulocyte hemoglobin content, erythrocyte ferritin and percent hypochromic RBC's but these are not currently universally available, nor do t hey necessarily offer any advantages over traditionally measures [14]. Once target iron stores are achieved, monitoring on a three to four month basis is required to avoid development of iron deficiency states and subsequent erythropoietin resistance.

Summary

Anemia is prevalent with patients with chronic kidney disease and is under-recognized resulting in under-treated. Commercially available recombinant human rHuEPO (Epoetin Alpa and Darbeopoetin Alpha) are available for treating this at risk population. Careful monitoring and replacement of iron is a necessary precursor to initiation of rHuEPO therapy. Targeting hemoglobins as recommended by the NKF K-DOQI workgroup has shown to positively impact this patient population as it pertains to quality of life measures, congestive heart failure, left ventricular hypertrophy and cognition. There are ongoing studies investigating various dosing regimen that target less frequent administration of recombinant human rHuEPO.

Robert Provenzano, M.D.
Division of Nephrology
Department of Internal Medicine
St John Hospital and Medical Center
Detroit, Michigan

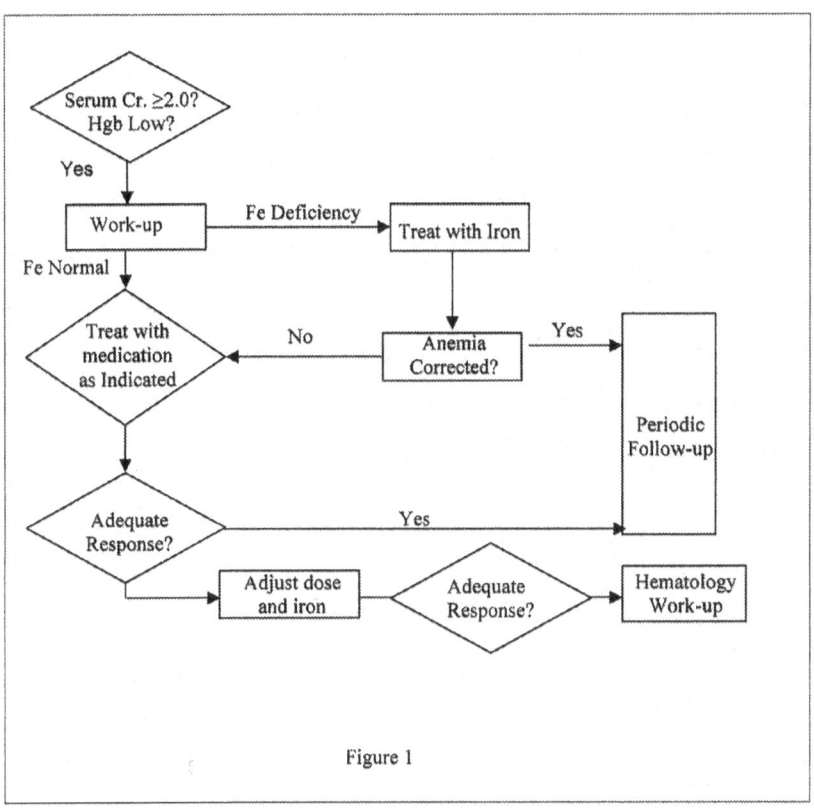

Figure 1

1.   Eschbach J, DeOreo P., Adamason, J. et al. RHuEPO clinical practice guidelines for the management of anemia of chronic renal failure. Am J Kidney Dis 1997;30:S192-240.

2.   Jones CA, McQuillan GM, Kusek, JQ, et al. Serum creatinine levels in the US population: Third National Health and Nutrition Examination Survey. Am J Kidney Dis 1998;32:992-999.

3.   Self KG, Conroy, MM, Eichner ER. Failure to diagnose anemia in medical inpatients. Is the traditional diagnosis of anemia a dying art ? Am J Med 1986;81: 786-790.

1.   Eschbach J, DeOreo P., Adamason, J. et al. RHuEPO clinical practice guidelines for the management of anemia of chronic renal failure. Am J Kidney Dis 1997;30:S192-240.

2.   Jones CA, McQuillan GM, Kusek, JQ, et al. Serum creatinine levels in the US population: Third National Health and Nutrition Examination Survey. Am J Kidney Dis 1998;32:992-999.

3.   Self KG, Conroy, MM, Eichner ER. Failure to diagnose anemia in medical inpatients. Is the traditional diagnosis of anemia a dying art? Am J Med 1986;81: 786-790.

4.   Collins A. Renal insufficiency intervention: Trends in anemia in the United States. ASN Satellite Symposium 2000.

5.   Kauz AT, Obrador GI, Pereira BJG. Anemia management in patients with chronic renal insufficiency. Am J Kidney Dis 2000;36 (suppl 3):S39-S51.

6.   Hakim RM, Lazarus JM. Biochemical parameters in chronic renal failure. Am J Kidney Dis 1988;11:238-247.

7.   7 Sarnak MJ, Levey AS. Cardiovascular disease and chronic renal disease: a new paradigm. Am J Kidney Dis 2000;35(suppl 1): S117-S131.

8.   Levin A. Prevalence of cardiovascular damage in early renal disease. Nephrol Dial transplant 2001;16(suppl s):7-11.

9.   Erslev AJ. Erythropoietin: Molecular, Cellular, and Clinical Biology. Baltimore, Md:Johns Hopkins University Press; 1991.

10.   Owen W. Clinical evaluation of once-weekly (QW) epoetin alpha dosing in patients (Pts) with anemia due to early renal insufficiency. J Am Soc Nephrol 2000; 10:Abst A0858.

11.   Provenzano R. Once-weekly treatment with epoetin alfa in patients with anemia due to chronic kidney disease: preliminary analysis. J Am Soc Nephrol 2001; 10:Abst 1227.

12.   Macdougall I, Tucker B, Thompson J. et al. A randomized controlled study of iron supplementation in patients treated with erythropoietin. Kidney Int 1996;50:1694-1699.

13. Feldman HI, Santanna J, Wensheng G, et al. Iron administration and clinical outcomes in hemodialysis patients. J Am Soc Nephrol 2002;13:734-744.

14. Goodnough LT, Skikne B, Brugnara C. Erythropoietin, irion, and erythropoiesis. Blood 2000;96:823-33.

15. NKF-DOQI Clinical Practice Guidelines for Anemia of Chronic Disease, 2000. Am J Kidney Dis 2001;37(suppl 1):S182-S238.

16. Eschbach JW, Egrie JC, Downing MR, et al. Correction of the anemia of end-stage renal disease with recombinant human erythropoietin: Results of a combined phase I and II clinical trial. N Engl J Med 1987;316:73-78.

17. Wingard RL, Parker RA, Ismail N, et al. Efficacy of oral iron therapy in patients receiving recombinant human erythropoietin. Am J Kidney Dis 1995;25:433-439.

Gender and Race Discrimination in US Uremia Therapy: What is The Truth?

Clinton D. Brown

INTRODUCTION

Before there was government funding, hemodialysis was rationed. A special committee appointed to review each case of end stage renal disease (ESRD) and determine who would receive the life saving treatment. Today a patient with ESRD has the option of receiving hemodialysis, chronic ambulatory peritoneal dialysis, or a kidney transplant (from a living relative or a cadaver) [1].

According to Medicare Law, all patients with ESRD are entitled to receive and must be offered the option of a renal transplant (as well as the option of either form of dialysis). In the case of African Americans the issues of renal failure and access to renal transplantation are complex. The first aspect of the problem is the concept of race. Is race a biologic construct or can it be defined purely in societal/cultural/environmental/historical terms? This question has sparked a great deal of controversy as the debates continue.

According to scholars [2,3], more than one constructs can be used to define race. The most conspicuous is race as a biologic entity (skin color, facial features, body habitus). This construct of race was a modern invention to categorize people who were perceived to be different (ie, others) and was used as a rationale for enslavement of indigenous people of American and Africa [4]. With the acceptance of race as a true and legitimate entity, blacks [in America] would endure a profound, permanent, and devastating alteration of their culture and history.

However, with the mapping of the human genome, scienteists concur that there is no biologic (genetic) bases for race. That not withstanding, there appears to be presentation or expression of medical disorders (frequency and severity) that are associated with certain populations. For example, keloid, the skin condition that results in excessive and occasionally painful scarring following trauma is seen almost exclusively in Africans and in the descendents of Africans [5]. The high proportion fo African American that develop ESRD is striking. Approximately 13% of the U.S. population is African American yet African American make up more than one third of all patients with ESRD [6].

As recent as the late nineties the incidence and prevalence of ESRD in African Americans was over four and five times, respectively, that in whites [7]. The reason(s) for the disproportionate representation of African Americans among those with ESRD h as not been elucidated. Some investigators believe that biologic variables such as over expression of transforming growth factor *Beta* [8], mutation of the angiotensin I-converting enzyme gene [9], or increased salt-sensitivity [10] make African Americans particularly vulnerable to renal failure.

Other investigators reject biologic mechanisms as an explanation for the high prevalence of ESRD in African American in favor of societal/cultural/environmental causes or causes attributed to race as a construct of ethnicity [11]. Lower socioeconomic class, lack of private health insurance [12], inappropriate treatment, poor communication between patient and health care professional, lack of sensitivity to cultural values and beliefs [13], are reasons why members of a disadvantaged minority group may not receive optimal health care. It is my belief that research that targets "racial"/biologic factors and ethnicity, will provide most useful information that will redress [serve to correct] the over representation of ESRD in African-Americans.

Access to Care

During the 1970's hemodialysis was the best option for renal replacement therapy. By the 1980's renal transplantation would be come the treatment which offered the highest quality of life, improved mortality,a nd shown to be the least costly over the long term [14]. Because of the benefits of renal transplantation, the federal government mandated that all patients developing ESRD be evaluated for a renal transplant.

In direct opposition to the intent of government's position on access to renal transplantation, are the reports of several authors bemoaning the less than equal allocation of transplants. Eggars reports that African Americans are only 37 percent as likely to receive a renal transplant [15, 1995]. Soucie et al, [16] reports that African American are far less likely to be identified as candidates for a renal transplant. Kasiske et al found that white patients are twice as likely to be placed on a renal transplant list as are African-Americans [12].

Finally, a prospective analysis of white and African-American patients with ESRD from four major geographic areas in the United States, found that whites who were medically suitable to have a transplant were five times likely to be transplanted than their African-American counterpart. Interestingly, 10 percent of white patients who were considered not medically suitable for transplantation received a renal transplant compared to 2 percent of African-American patients who were similarly not medically suitable to undergo transplantation. The authors concluded that renal transplantation was over utilized in whites and under utilized in African-Americans [17].

The racial differences in renal transplantation may be explained in part by criteria base don immunologic mechanisms [18]. However, social issues play a major role in the early phases of the complex process of transplantation.

Institutionalized Racism

The oppressive system which began as a rationale for economic exploitation of African and their descendants promoted exclusions of rights, opportunity, goods, services, power, social responsibility, and denied access to life choices and health care. With the passage of time and government intervention, the system of overt racial discrimination evolved to become subtle, covert system of operation [institutionalized racism] that is fueled by pervasive ideologies and perceptions of minority people.

According to some scholars, institutional racism may exist even when individuals who make decisions for social structures (ie, health care, education, law) might intend no racial prejudice or without the victim being aware that racism exist. The systemic operations of an institution which controls opportunity for employment, promotion, criteria for merit, social ideologies, and the interdependence of social institutions (education, law, health care) are important determinants of equity in society rather than the actions of biased individuals. However, the actions of individuals who have decision-making –authority (in the case of renal transplantation—physicians and other health care providers, health society consultants) who subscribe to traditional behavior and rules regarding race related issues should not be minimized.

For example, some health professionals believe that minority patients are better off opting for hemodialysis rather than the superior choice of renal transplantation. Lowe et al's [19], stunning account of an Australian nephrologist's attitude toward an indigenous Australian woman who recently developed ESRD illustrates this point. The nephrologist dissuaded the patient from receiving a kidney transplant from her sister. The action taken by the nephrologist was explained by the quote: 'these people don't do well with transplants'.

Another problem facing health care providers when serving minority patients is the history of overt exploitation, mistreatment and misinformation. Understandable, the health care professional may be viewed by the African American patient as one who represents the elitist medical/health care system. When members of an African American community were surveyed on the subject of organ donation some of the reasons for their reluctance to grant permission for organ donation were: distrust of the medical establishment, fear of premature declaration of death if a donor card was signed, and a lack of awareness of organ transplantation [20].

Solutions

Institutional racism has its largest impact early in the transplantation process. However, institutional racism need not be a permanent social condition. It is dynamic by nature and will change as a result of social pressure (ie, public outcry, local protest, political movement, government mandate, empowerment of minority communities).

For more than two decades efforts to increase awareness of kidney transplantation and organ donation in minority communities throughout the United States have been extremely successful [20]. Spearheaded by the noted transplant surgeon, Dr Clive Callender, the success of this education program is attributed to the face to face grass root approach in which trained educators/coordinators, African American donor families, and transplant recipieints, expose community people to the facts about transplantation. Support from the private and government sectors, and collaboration with local organizations and transplant programs also contribute to the programs overall success.

CONCLUSIONS

As stated earlier, racial disparity in renal transplantation is a complex problem. Its correction will require intervention and change on many fronts: 1) an intense research initiative to root out and fix the biologic (immunologic) and nonbiologic causes of kidney failure in African American people, 2) training/retraining of health care professionals to achieve cultural competency, 3) continued organ transpolant educational campaigns in minority communities, and 4) extension of government funding for immunosuppression medication beyond the current period of three years.

Clinton D. Brown, M.D.
Renal Disease Division
SUNY Downstate Medical Center, Brooklyn, New York

REFERENCES

1. Held PJ, Pauly MV, Bovbjerg, Newmann J, Salvatierra O. Access to kidney transplantation. Ach Intern Med .1988;148: 2594-2600.
2. Herman AA. Towaed a Conceptualization of race in epidemiologic research. Ethnicity & Disease. 1996;6:7-20.
3. King G. Institutional racism and the medical/health complex: A conceptual analysis. Ethnicity & Disease. 1996;6:30-43.
4. Goldberg DT. Racist Culture: Philosophy and the politics of meaning. Cambridge, MA:Blackwell Publishers, 1993, pp61-89.
5. Dustan HP. Does keloid pathogenesis hold the key to understanding black/white differences in hypertension severity? Hypertension. 1995;26:858-62.
6. Young CJ and Gaston RS.Renal Transplantation in black Americans. N Engl J Med. 2000;343:1545-52.
7. Cecka JM. UNOS Scientific Renal Transplant Registry-2000. Clin Transpl, 2000:1-8.
8. Suthanthiran M, Khanna A, Cukran D. Transforming growth factor beta, hyperexpression in African-American end-stage renal disese patients. Kidney Int. 1998;53:639-4.
9. Bloem LJ, Manatunga AK, Pratt JH. Racial difference in the relationship of an angiotensin I-converting enzyme activity. Hypertension. 1996;27:62-6.
10. Powers DR, Wallin JD. End-stage renal disease in specific ethnic and racial groups: risk factors and benefits of antihypertensive therapy. Arch Intern Med. 1998;158:793-800.
11. Kiefe CI. Race/Ethnicity and cancer survival. JAMA. 2002;287: 2138-9.
12. Kasiske BL, London W, Ellison MD. Race and socioeconomic factors influencing early placement on the Kidney transplant waiting list. J Am Soc Nephol. 1998;9: 2142-7.
13. Klassen AC, Hall AG, Saksvig B, et al. Relationship between patients' perceptions of disadvantage and discrimination and listing for kidney transplantation. Am J Public Health. 2001;92:811-17.
14. Eggers PW.Comparison of treatment costs between dialysis and

transplantation. Seminars in Nephrology. 1992;12:284-9.

15. Eggers PW. Racial differences in access to kidney transplantation. Health Care Fin Rev.1995;89-103.

16. Soucie JM, Neylan JF, McClelllan W. Race and sex differences in he indentification of candidates for renal transplantation. Am J Kidney Dis. 1992;19:414-9.

17. Epstein AM, Ayanian JZ, Keogh JH, et al.Racial disparites in access to renal transplantation. 2000;343:1537-44.

18. Sanfilippo FP, Vaughn WK, Peters TG, et al. Factors affecting the waiting time for cadaveric kidney transplant candidates in the United States. JAMA. 1992;267;247-52.

19. Lowe M, Kerridge IH, Mitchell KR. 'These sorts of people don't do very well': race and allocation of health care resources. J of Medical Ethics1991;211:——

20. Callender C, Hall LE, Yeager CL, Dunston et al. Organ donation and Blacks. A critical frontier. N Engl J Med, 1992;325:442-4.

Strategies to Maximize Organ Donation in the Inner City

Clive O. Callendar, MD, Patrice V. Miles, Margruetta B. Hall, Ph.D.

Introduction

The National Minority Organ Tissue Transplant Education Program (MOTTEP) is the actualization of 15 years of systematic study and research beginning in 1980 to investigate the low rate of organ donation among the Black population. Members of the Southeastern Organ Procurement Foundation (SEOPF) approached Dr. Clive Callender to evaluate data they had recently reviewed which stated that 50% to 70% of all dialysis patients listed with the Foundation were black, yet less than 10% of the organ donors at that time were black [1].

Armed with a $500 grant from Howard University Hospital, two 2-hour focus group sessions were convened with 40 black residents of Washington, DC. These focus group sessions identified the five obstacles to donation within the Black community. They were:

1. Lack of awareness about transplantation.
2. Religious myths and misperceptions (superstitions).
3. Distrust of the medical community.
4. Fear of premature death.
5. Racism.

When the focus group session began, only two of the forty persons had signed donor cards. After the session, all forty participants signed donor cards. It was concluded that having face-to face dialogue with persons such as transplant recipients, transplant candidates, donors and donor family members providing personal testimonies, along with healthcare professionals, was the key to changing attitudes towards donation. In addition to the grass-roots strategy, the mass media was enlisted to assist in the awareness process. A 50 city media tour was sponsored by Dow Chemical Company beginning in 1986. The number of persons becoming highly aware of organ donation increased from 10% in 1985 to 35% in 1990 [2].

What Does National MOTTEP Do?

Based on the aforementioned, National MOTTEP was established in 1991 and applies the same methodology of face-to-face dialogue to all ethnic minority populations. Upon National MOTTEP's inception, the program's overall goal was to increase the number of minority donors. However, due to the alarming rate of increase in persons being added to the waiting list (1989 = 16,000 vs. 2001 77,000) versus those actually receiving transplants (2001 = 21,000), National MOTTEP revised its mission to reduce the rate and numbe rof ethnic minority Americans needing organ and tissue transplants. The program targets African American, Hispanic/Latino, Asian, Pacific Islander, Native American and Alaska Native populations. National MOTTEP has targeted these populations within 15 major cities across the country.

National MOTTEP has broadened its efforts of changing the level of knowledge, attitudes and behaviors by incorporating several approaches. Utilizing community volunteers and messengers who reside within the respective target areas and are ethnically similar and culturally sensitive has been crucial and effective. The number of volunteers has increased from 60 in 1995 to vero 500 as of 2001. The approaches include:

1.   Community participation and direction – Encourages the involvement of persons in the planning and implementation of their own activities.
2.   Face-to-face presentations – Making presentations at schools, social, civic and religious events.
3.   Collaboration and partnerships – Collaborating with community based organizations to promote the program's mission and goals.
4.   Media promotion – Utilizing media (radio, television and print) in the positive promotion of organ/tissue donation.

5. Information dissemination – Developing culturally sensitive and informative brochures, flyers, fact sheets and other information.
6. Evaluation – Developing comprehensive quantitative and qualitative surveys to gauge the effectiveness of its programs [3].

In a further exploration of community participation and direction, National MOTTEP's volunteers have assisted in the planning of community awareness activities such as Golf Tournaments, Dance for life, Candlelight Vigils and a Multicultural Fashion Show. Through these types of activities, more than 6 million persons have been reached. Because it is also a goal to educate youth about donation as well as preventive health to prevent the need for transplantation in future years, youth specific activities have been implemented such as Teen Health Summits, Poster Contests, and a Mascot Contest. These activities have reached more than 83,000 youth [3].

As National MOTTEP has established programs within the various ethnic minority communities, the research reveals that the obstacles and barriers are consistent with those identified with the Black community in 1980.

Hispanic/Latino Obstacles: Lack of access to medical care, language and economic barrier to medical care, lack of transplant awareness, fear of premature death, religious and cultural beliefs, distrust of doctors and the medical system and racism.

Asian and Pacific Islander Obstacles (Filipino population): Fear of death, cultural beliefs, keeping the body in tact and undisturbed after death, mistrust of the medical community, fear of premature death and religious beliefs.

Alaska Native Obstacles: Lack of awareness and distrust of the medical system.

Native American Obstacles: Various tribal beliefs regarding death and organ donation, strong taboo surrounding death, religious beliefs, and keeping the body whole [4].

Why Is Prevention Necessary and Why is National MOTTEP Addressing the Prevention Component?

1. While minority donation rates have increased since 1980 and minorities are donating at a percentage equal to or greater than their respective population distribution, due to the waiting times (an average of 3-5 years for kidney transplants), more minority donors are needed.

2. Minorities wait twice as long for transplants than their white counterparts.

3. Minorities represent more than 50% of those waiting for kidney transplants.

4. Every 14 minutes a new name is added to the national waiting list.

5. 12 persons die each day awaiting a life saving transplant.

6. Billions of dollars could be saved in health care costs.

National MOTTEP is the first national transplant related program to address the shortage of donors using a two-fold strategy – increasing the number of donors while decreasing the number of persons who need transplants. All community activities address both areas. The target audiences have become more receptive to donation (intervention) when the dialogue includes taking care of self as the priority (prevention). While donation is about saving lives, lives are also being saved through prevention. The prevention components include hypertension, diabetes, alcohol and substance abuse, nutrition and exercise.

The results of National MOTTEP's mission emphasizing both prevention and intervention are:

1. Healthier lifestyles and behavioral patterns.
2. Increased number of minority donors and transplant recipients.

3. Increased number of family discussions regarding organ and tissue transplants.
4. Increased number of minority donor pledges.

Although, the topic of prevention is mentioned repeatedly, the overall goal is still addressing the donor shortage that continues to be the number one problem in transplantation.

What Has National MOTTEP Accomplished?

As previously stated, the evaluation component gauges the effectiveness of the program. National MOTTEP's evaluation component is designed to: 1) assess the extent to which minorities are being educated about organ/tissue donation and transplantation; 2) assess the level of increase of organ/tissue donations after MOTTEP presentations; and 3) determine whether target populations intend to change their health behavior practices to prevent the need for transplantation [4].

In addition to a pre-intervention and post intervention questionnaire administered during formal heatlh presentations, participants are also asked to participate in a 2-6 month follow-up telephone study. Major question areas are: Did they signed a donor card? Did they have a family discussion about donation? Were they willing to be an organ/tissue donor? Did they need more information on the subject? and Did they change any health habits since the presentation?

Initial findings indicated the following:
*   • 57% signed donor cards by the time the follow-up interview was held, compared with 36% who stated that they had signed donor cards before attending a MOTTEP presentation; and
*   • 62% reported having family discussions by the time of the follow-up interview, compared to 40% reporting that they had family discussions before attending a MOTTEP presentation [5].

Summary

In conclusion, it is very clear that community involvement, education and empowerment are key elements in solving the donor shortage and changing health behaviors. It is absolutely essential to educate the community on the continuing need for organ/tissue donors (living and cadaveric), the donation process, and the diseases and behaviors which lead to the need for transplantation [5]. Each individual within target communities holds the key for taking responsibility for a

problem in which there is an easy solution. Making the right decision. Saying yes to donation as well as agreeing to change health habits in order to live a more healthy and prosperous life and preventing the need for transplantation in the first place.

Clive O. Callender, M.D., F.A.C.S.
Transplant Center
Department of Surgery
Howard University Hospital
Washington, DC

References

1.   Callender CO. The results of transplantation in blacks: just the tip of the iceberg. Transplantation Proc 1989;21:3407-3410.
2.   Reitz NN, Callender CO. Organ donation in the African-American population: a fresh perspective with a simple solution. N Natl Med Assoc 1993;85(5):353-8.
3.   Callender, CO, Miles, PV. Obstacles or organ donation in ethnic minorities. Pediatr Transplant 2001;5: 383-385.
4.   Callender CO, Miles PV, Hall MB. National MOTTEP: educating to prevent the need for transplantation. Minority Organ Tissue Transplant Education Program. Ethn Dis 2002;12(1):S1-34-7.
5.   Callendar CO, Hall MB, Branch D. An assessment of the effectiveness of the Mottep model for increasing donation rates and preventing the need for transplantation—adult findings: program years 1998 and 1999. Semin Nephrol 2001;21(4):419-28.

Hyperlipidemia in Kidney Disease: Effects on Disease Progression and Mortality

T.L. Nickolas, A.S. Appel, G.B. Appel

Introduction

Patients with the nephritic syndrome, renal insufficiency, and those on dialysis or status-post transplantation all have different patterns of lipid abnormalities. Cardiovascular disease is the major cause of mortality and a major contributor to morbidity in all forms of renal disease [1-4]. Although there is less data available on patients with the nephritic syndrome or mild to moderate renal insufficiency, the data on cardiovascular mortality and morbidity for the ESRD population is compelling. The percentage of new patients with diabetes in the ESRD population has increased from 30% in 1988 to over 40% in the late 1990's to over 50% in the new millennium [5].

The mortality rate of the ESRD population directly correlates with the age of the patient, and diabetics have the highest mortality rates of all common ESRD conditions [3,6]. The leading cause of death of all ESRD patients in all age groups over 20 years old is CVD. The total percent of deaths due to CVD (cardiac arrest, acute myocardial infarction, cerebrovascular disease, and other cardiac deaths) is almost 50% for these patents 20-44 years old, AND OVER 55% for patients OVER 45 years old. The CVD mortality is even higher for diabetic patients on hemodialysis and peritoneal dialysis [3,6]. The CVD mortality in transplant patients remains high as well.

There is little doubt that lipid abnormalities contribute to the high risk of cardiovascular disease seen in these populations. A more controversial question has focused on whether dyslipidemia itself contributes to renal damage. For over 100 years it has been suggested that hyperlipidemia worsens renal disease. In 1982 Moorhead et al proposed that lipid abnormalities may

126

contribute to its progression, but the data were inconclusive [7].

Recent data from animal models, uncontrolled and controlled clinical trials of the relationship of dyslipidemia to renal progression, and a major meta-analysis of the effects of anti-hyperlipidemics on renal progression all support the concept that lipid abnormalities not only independently contribute to the progression of established renal disease, but may also contribute to the initiation of renal disease.

Evidence from Animal Models

Animal models of renal disease have examined the correlation between lipid abnormalities and athe course of renal disease. These include animals with endogenous hyperlipidemia and animals fed hyperlipidemic diets. The effects on these animals of lipid lowering agents have also been studied [8]. Thus, in rats, guinea pigs,a dn rabbits fed lipogenic diets, focal glmerulosclerosis develops [9,10]. Endogenous hyperlipidemia in the obese Zucker rat is also associated with progressive glomerulosclerosis and albuminuria [11].

Lipid lowering medications of entirely different classes (clofibrate and HMG-COA reductase inhibitors) have led to lowered plasma cholesterol levels and less albuminuria and glomerulosclerosis in these models. In some models this effect has been shown to be unrelated to alterations of glomerular hemodynamics [12]. The potential mechanism(s) whereby lipid abnormalities lead to progressive renal disease are still being defined. Experimental data suggest that there are many similarities between glomerulosclerosis and the atherosclerotic process [13,14]. Mesangial cells share many properties with vascular smooth muscle cells and take up both unaltered and oxidized LDL cholesterol [15]. Under hyperlipemic conditions, LDL in the mesangial matrix can undergo oxidation. This can result in uptake via scavenger receptors on mesangial cells and monocyte-macrophages. Oxidized LDL, lipid peroxides, and lysolipids of oxidized LDL can act as cytotoxic agents on mesangial, epithelial,a nd endothelial cells, thereby contributing to cell damage and sclerosis, associated in some in vitro studies with proliferation and death of mesangial cells [15]. Damage to endothelial cells can cause monocyte adherence and platelet aggregation on the endothelium. In some models, intraglomerular hemodynamics may be altered by the lipid abnormalities [16].

Other models have suggested that tubulointerstitial damage can occur from hyperlipedmia [17], even without primary glomerular disease [17,18]. In these experiments renal mRNA for transforming growth factor-B1 (TGF-B1) and the chemokine, monocyte chemoattractant protein-1 (MCP-1), were elevated and believed to be involved in the pathologic changes.

The Role of Lipids in Human Renal Disease

Despite animal evidence indicating that dyslipidemia can initiate renal disease, data in humans are scarce. Only a few studies have examined whether lipids are associated with progressive renal disease in populations with no or minimal renal dysfunction. The Helsinki Heart Study (HHS) examined a subset of 2700 males with elevated non-HDL cholesterol levels and found that low HDL cholesterol predicted a progressive rise in serum creatinine. This was true in both patients taking an antihyperlipidemic medication (gemfibrozil) and those on placebo. Moreover, the correlation between low HDL cholesterol and rise in serum creatinine was even greater than that for the relationship between hypertension and progressive renal disease. Triglyceride levels were unrelated to a rise in serum creatinine [19].

A second study, the Atherosclerosis Risk in Communities Study (ARIC), examined the relationship between plasma lipids and a rise in serum creatinine of 0.4 mg/dl in 12,700 patients with baseline creatinine <2.0 mg/dl in males and <1.8 mg/dl in females. At almost three years of follow-up 191 of the patients had a rise in the creatinine, for an incidence of 5.1/1000 patient years. After adjustment for race, gender, age, presence of diabetes, initial serum creatinine, hypertension, and use of antihypertensive medications, patients with elevated triglycerides and lower HDL (especially HDL2) cholesterol at baseline were at significantly increased risk for progressive renal disease. The risk was greater for higher tertiles of elevated triglycerides and for lower tertiles of HDL cholesterol. It was significant even for patients with normal levels of baseline serum creatinine and for both diabetics and non-diabetics [20].

A number of studies have looked at whether dyslipidemia contributes to the progression of renal disease in patients with established renal dysfunction. One study by Samuelsson et al prospectively followed a population of 73 adult non-diabetic patients with primary renal disease for an average of 3.2 years. The majority (43/73) of the patients had chronic glomerulonephritis as the etiology of their kidney disease, and baseline GFR was 41 ml/min/

1.73 m2 BSA. Elevated total cholesterol, LDL cholesterol, and especially apollipoprotein B were all significantly related to a more rapid decline in renal function over time while HDL cholesterol and triglycerides were not. The average rate of GFR decline was 2.8 ml/min/1.73 m2 annually. In the chronic glomerulonephritis patients the association was more significant, and triglycerides and apolipoprotein E levels were also correlated with progression. Although the presence of proteinuria and hypertension were both related to progression, the data suggest these factors were independent and compounding. Thus, proteinuria and hypercholesterolemia each contributed to the decline in GFR [21].

In the Modification of Diet in Renal Disease (MDRD) study, an analysis of 840 patients with renal diseases of different causes and severities, 6 factors that independently predicted a faster decline in GFR or which altered the efficacy of diet or blood pressure interventions were identified. Patients in this study had GFRs ranging from 13 to 55 mL/min/1.73m2 and were followed for up to 3.5 years. The patients were stratified into 2 groups according to a GFR of either 13 to 24 mL/min/1.73m2 or 25 to 55 mL/min/1.73m2. The independent factors included greater urinary protein excretion, a diagnosis of polycystic kidney disease, lower serum transferring, higher mean arterial pressure, black race, and lower serum HDL cholesterol. Lower HDL cholesterol affected the rate of GFR decline in only the higher baseline GFR group [22].

Although there have been a number of small studies in diabetics and non-diabetics that evaluated the effect of anati-hyperlipidemic therapy on the course of renal disease progression, most have been too small to draw clear conclusions. A recent meta-analysis reviewed 13 prospective controlled trials from 1991 through 1999 examining over 260 patients followed for at least 3 months. In t his meta-analysis the mean age was 49 yeares old, and over 60 % of patients were male. Of the studies 7 dealt with diabetic patients, 3 with glomerulonephritis and others were unspecified. All but two dealth with "statin" therapy. The results showed a lower rate of decline in GFR with antihyperlipidemic therapy versus controls. The effect did not correlate with study design or quality, percentage change in cholesterol, type of renal disease, or type of antihyperlipidemic medication. Patients with a longer follow up duration had a greater effect of slowing the progression than patients followed for a shorter duration of time. There was also a trend towards a favorable effect on proteinuria and albumin excretion with anithyperlipidemic therapy but heterogeneity of studies prevent clear conclusions in this area [23].

The Role of Statins

The role of lipid lowering therapy on the effects of hyperlipidemia is just being realized. Aside from lowering lipid levels, agents such as HMG-Co A reductase inhibitors may have many other beneficial effects on the glomerulus. In experimental models, they may suppress cell proliferation, inhibit activation of transcription factors (NFkB), block intracellular mitogen stimulated signaling pathways, improve vascular hemodynamics via alterations of nitric oxide, and reduce platelet aggregation [24-27]. In some experimental situations, the effects of the "statins" have been independent of teir lipid lowering effect, while in others there has been an association of both effects making mechanistic conclusions about the role of the lipids themselves difficult. For example, in several animal models, an HMG-CoA reductase inhjibitor has led to improvement in renal hemodynamics, increased renal blood flow, and GFR preservation [28]. In these animal models the effects were independent of cholesterol lowering although probably dependent upon interference with mevalonate pathways withint he kidney or vasculature [29,30]. In a recent double-blind cross-over human study of ten patients with autosomal dominant polycystic kidney disease only four week sof therapy with simvastatin led to improvement in GFR and effective renal plasma flow. These effects were associated with an enhanced vasodilator response to acetylcholine in the forearm that was mediated by nitric oxide and attenuated by a nitric oxide synthase inhibitor. Although cholesterol and lipid fractions were significantly reduced by the statin therapy, the actual effects on renal function are more likely to be mediated by direct effects of the statin on mevalonate pathways involved in endothelial function. [31].

Conclusions

Dyslipidemia is common in many forms of renal disease and certainly contributes to atherosclerotic complications and morbidity in these diseases. Although in the past animal data and some human studies have suggested a role for dyslipidemia in the progression of renal failure, the data have been far from conclusive. Recent uncontrolled studies, controlled trials, and a meta-analysis of the effects of antihyperlipidemics all provide strong evidence that lipids may contribute to renal progression and that lipid lowering agents may slow this progression. Although many of the studies deal with HMG-CoA reductase inhibitors which have many actions beyond their antihyperlipidemic effect, the fact that other antihyperlipidemics have been beneficial and the positive correlations in populations with mild renal disease and without lipid-lowering therapy reinforce the conclusion that dyslipidemia does indeed contribute to progressive renal disease.

Gerald B. Appel, M.D.
Nephrology Division
Department of Medicine
Columbia University College of Physicians & Surgeons
New York, New York

References

1.   Sarnak MJ, Levey AS. Cardiovascular Disease and Chronic Renal Disease: A New Paradigm Am J Kidney Dis 2000;35 S117-S131.
2.   AHA. Heart and Stroke Statistical Update, 1998.
3.   Foley RN, Parfrey PS, Sarnak MJ. The clinical epidemiology of cardiovascular disease in chronic renal disease. Am J Kidney Dis 1998;32:S112-S119.
4.   Curtis BM, Parfrey PS. How can the cardiac death rate be reduced in dialysis patients? semin Dial 2002;15(1):22-4.
5.   US Renal Data Systems 1999 Annual Data Report. Bethesda Md NIH, NIDDK1999.
6.   Herzog CA, Ma JZ, Collins AJ. Poor long-term survival after myocardial infarction among patients on long term hemodialysis. N Eng J Med 1998;339:799-805.
7.   Moorehead JF, Chan MK, El Nahas M, Varghese Z. Lipied nephrotoxicity in chronic progressive glomerular and tubulointerstitial disease. Lancet 1982; a:1309-1311.
8.   Kamanna VS, Roh DD, Kirschenbaum MA. Hyperlipidemia and kidney disease: concepts derived from histopathology and cell biology of the glomerulus. Histol Histopathol 1998;13(1):169-179.
9.   Eddy AA. Interstitial fibrosis in hypercholesterolemic rats: role of oxidation, matrix synthesis,a nd proteolytic cascades. Kidney Int 1998;53 (5):1182-1189.
10.   Kasiske BL, O'Donnell MP, Schmitz PG, Kim Y&, Keane WF. Renal injury of diet-induced hypercholesterolemia in rats. Kidney Int 1990;37(3):880-891.
11.   Kamanna VS, Kirschenbaum MA. Association between very-low-density lipoprotein and glomerular injury in Zucker rats. Am J Nephrol 1993;13 (1):53-8.
12.   Grone EF, Walli AK, Grone HJ, Miller, Seidel D. The role of lipids in nephrolosclerosis and glomerulosclerosis. Atherosclerosis 1994;107(1):1-13.
13.   Diamond J, Karnovsky M. Focal and segmental glomerulosclerosis: Analogies to atherosclerosis. Kidney Int 1988;33:917-924.

14. Avram MM. Similarities between glomerular sclerosis and athersclerosis in human renal biopsy specimens: a role for lipoprotein glomerulopathy. Am J Med 1989; 87 (5N): 39N-41N.

15. Schlondorff D. Cellular mechanisms of lipid injury in the glomerulus. Am J Kidney Dis 1993;22(1):72-82.

16. Fuiano G, Esposito C, Sepe V, Colucci G, Bovino M, Rosa M, BallettaM, Bellinghieri G, Conte G, Cianciaruso B, Canton A. Effects of hypercholesterolemia of renal hemodynamics: study in patients with nephritic syndrome. Nephron 1996;73 (3): 430-435.

17. Grone HJ, Hohback J, Grone EF. Modulation of glomerular sclerosis and intersititial fibrosis by native and modified lipoproteins. Kidney Int Suppl 1996; 54:S18-22.

18. Eddy AA, McCulloch L, Liu E, Adams J. A relationship between proteinuria and acute tubgulointerstitial disease in rats with experimental nephritic syndrome. Am J Pathol 1991;138 (5):1111-1123.

19. Manttari M, Tiula E, AlikoskiT, Manninen V. Effects of hypertension and dyslipidemia on the decline in renal function. Hypertension 1995;26:670-676.

20. Muntner P, Coresh J, Smith JC, Eckfeldt J, Klang MJ. Plasma Lipids and risk of developing renal dysfunction: the atherosclerosis risk in communities study. Kidney Int 2000;58:293-301.

21. Samuelsson O, Mulec H, Knight-Gibson C, Atman PO, Kron B, Larsson R, Weiss L, Wedel H, Alaupovic P. Lipoprotein abnormalities are associated with increased rate of progression of human chronic renal insufficiency. Nephrol Dial Transplant 1997;12:1908-1915.

22. Hunsicker LG, Adler S, Caggiula A, England BK, Greene T, Kusek JW, Rogers NL, Teschan PE. Predictors of the progression of renal disease in the Modification of Diet in renal Disease Study. Kidney Int 1997;51 (6):1908-19.

23. Fried LF, Orchard TJ, Kasiske BL. Effect of lipid reduction on the progression of renal disease: a meta-analysis. Kidney Int 2001;59: 260-269.

24. Keane WF, Kasiske BL, O'Donnell MP, Kim Y. The role of altered metabolism in the progression of renal disease: experimental evidence. Am J Kidney Dis 1991;17 (Suppl 1):38-42.

25. Guijarro C, Kim Y, Schnoover CM, Massy ZA, O'Donnell MP,

Kasiske BL, Keane WF, Kashtan CE. Lovastatin inhibits NK-kB activation in human mesangial cells. Nephrol Dial Transplant 1996;11:990-996.

26.   Kim SY, Guijarro C, O'Donnell MP, Kasiske BL, Kim Y, Keane WF. Human mesangial cell production of monocye chemoattractant protein-1: modulation by lovastatin. Kidney Int. 1995;48:363-371.

27.   Miyazaki K, Isbel NM, Lan HY, Hattroi M, Ito K, Bbacher M, Bucala R, Atkins RC, Nikolic Paterson DJ. Up-regulation oc macrophage colony stimulating factor (M-CSF) and migration inhibitory factor (MIF) expression and monocyte recruitment during lipid-induced glomerular injury in the exogenous hypercholesterolemic rat (ExHC). Clin Exp Immunol 1997;108:318-323.

28.   Jiang J, Sun CW, Alonsogalicia N, Roman RJ. Lovastatin reduces renal vascular reactivity in spontaneously hypertensive rats. Am J Hypertens 1998;11:1222-1231.

29.   Stroes E, Koomans H, de Bruin T, Rabelink T. Vascular function in the forearm of hypercholerterolemic patients off and on lipid-lowering medication. Lancet 1995;346:467-471.

30.   O'Driscoll G, Green D, Taylor RR. Simvastatin, an HMG-coenzyme A reductase inhibitor, improves endothelial function witin 1 month. Circulation 1997;95:1126-1131.

31.   van Dijk MA, Kamper AM, van Veen S, Souverijn JHM, Blauw GJ. Effect of simvastatin on renal function in autosomal dominant polycystic kidney disease. Nephrol Dial Transplant 2001;16:2152-2157.

Do For-Profit Dialysis Companies Care More About Profits Than Patients?

Neil R. Powe and Edwina Young

INTRODUCTION

Over the past decade, the number of for-profit End Stage Renal Disease care providers have steadily increased in the United States, while the number of non-profit providers have remained relatively consistent. In 1990 only about 1,100 facilities were for-profit. This number has nearly tripled to 2,900 and presently, only about a quarter of all the providers of ESRD care in the US remains non-profit. (Figure I). Consolidation by for-profit providers has also arisen rapidly. Now a relatively small number of companies treat a large proportion of the population of dialysis patients with Gambro Healthcare, Total Renal Care, and Fresenius as the top three for-profit providers with regard to patient volume.

Both for profit and not profit facilities increasingly struggle against rising dialysis care costs because dialysis reimbursement has remained the static since 1974. In fact, there is a steadily decreasing reimbursement rate after adjustment for inflation. (Figure II) This has put immense pressure for dialysis providers to cut costs and raise efficiency. The increasing number of for-profit facilities, and in particular publically traded companies, suggest that for-profit units may achieve efficiencies in providing care through the use of corporate business practices and infusion of resources for improved technology. Implicitly investors in such units believe they will reap financial rewards.

One strategy for survival in the face of economic pressures is to maintain income through high patient volume. One study found that for-profit sole proprietorship dialysis facilities provide an average of 146 more treatments per month than a comparable non-profit facilities for the same labor, capital and supply inputs [1]. However, there have also been concerns about the impact of extreme efficiency on quality of care in ESRD patients because a growing body of evidence suggests that ownership may influence decisions and patient outcomes. Some speculate that under a constrained, capitated reimbursement for care, efforts to maintain income and patient volume compromise quality of care. The logic put forth is that for profit organizations may be more sensitive than their non profit counterparts to these economic pressures.

Quality of Care

The relationship between quality of care and facility ownership has been studied using the Donabedian model of evaluation of the quality of care. Donabedian's model evaluates the quality of care by examining three important aspects: structure, process, and outcomes. (Figure III)

Structure — Structure pertains to components of the facility such as staffing, location, and equipment. Research into the structure of dialysis facilities has resulted in findings of significant differences between non-profit and for-profit organizations. Average patient to staff ratios of for-profit facilities may be higher than for non-profit facilities, 4.86 patients per staff member versus 3.88 patients per staff member, respectively – an average difference of approximately one more patient per care member in for-profit facilities than in non-profit facilities [2]. The composition of the staff also differs between the two ownership types. Non-profit facilities appear to have a higher ratio of administrators with clinical training than non-profit facilities [3]. In addition, 40% of for-profit administrators only underwent business training, compared to the 14% of non-profit administrators who did likewise. The policies carried out by each facility could have an influence on patient care and reflect the differences in the training of its administrators.

Process – The processes of care are the tasks performed in providing care. These includes aspects such as modality selection, dialysis dosing practices, dialyzer re-use practices and medication use practices. A study of the views of facility administrators suggests that administers vary with regard to the processes of care they implement under certain situations. Given a hypothetical increase in Medicare reimbursement, both for profit and not for profit administrators share the view of improving patient education as

136

first choice of where to allocate increased funding [3]. Nevertheless, there are some differences by ownership. For-profit administrators tend to also favor policies of increasing returns to investors and raising staff salaries. Also, given a decrease in reimbursement, for profit administrators would return less to investors, decrease hours of operation, close a facility, and limit staff salaries more often than not for profit administrators.

There are other differences in process of care between non-profit and for-profit facilities. Dialyzer re-use, a practice now used by both non-profit and for-profit facilities as a means of lowering costs, was earlier more often used in for-profit than in not for profit facilities [4]. Also, evidence from the United States Renal Data System suggests that a higher proportion of non-profit facility patients receives flu and pneumonia vaccines and lipid monitoring [5]. For-profit facilities, on the other hand, appear to provide glycosylated hemoglobin testing to more patients.

The differences in ways that for profit and not for profit administrators respond to reimbursement changes is illustrated by the introduction of recombinant human erythropoietin in the late 1980s. In June 1989, Medicare approved payment for recombinant human erythropoietin therapy at 80% of an allowed charge of $40 for up to 10,000 units provided to an anemic dialysis patient. This payment mechanism provided a financial incentive to administer low doses. Medicare subsequently raised their reimbursement rate in January 1991 to include a variable payment per treatment of $11 per 1000 units.

A study comparing recombinant human erythropoietin dosing in dialysis patients before and after the implement of this policy showed that facilities respond to financial incentives and that they vary in their response by ownership type [5]. This cohort study of 29,088 patients compared ownership effects on the dosing of recombinant human erythropoietin showed that average doses of patieints receiving erythropoietin were lower than those in clinical trials under the fixed payment scheme of $40 for administration of up to 10,000 units of erythropoietin. All facilities (except for government affiliated) raised their treatment doses over six months after the revision ofhte Medicare payment. However, the change in dose was greater in for-profit than in not for profit facilities. These results strongly suggested that for-profit facilities respond to a greater degree to reimbursement incentives than non-profit facilities.

Outcomes – Differences in process of care can translate into differences in outcomes including survival, morbidity quality of life and patient satisfaction. Another cohort study has elucidated the relationship between ownership and outcomes [6]. Using data from the US Renal Data System special studies and USRDS/HCFA administrative data, this cohort study focused on the two patient outcomes of survival and referral for transplantation.

This study found that mortality was greater for patients treated in for profit versus not for profit facilities (Figure IV). It also found that the rates of placement on waiting lists for a kidney transplant were lower among patients treated at for-profit versus non –profit facilities. Because kidney transplantation results in better quality and logner length of life for dialysis patients, placement on the waiting list can be thought of as a proximate indicator of outcome. Other studies have subsequently corroborated that such mortality differences exist [7,8]. The study additionally explored the potential effect of competitive forces on these outcomes. For-profit facilities located in an area without non-profit facilities had accentuated negative outcomes suggesting that quality-based competition may occur in dialysis markets where both types of facilities operate (Figure V).

Organizational Missions and Quality of Care

These differences in process and outcomes suggest that different types of dialysis facilities may have different missions. However, the following excerpts from mission statements of dialysis organizations indicate that quality of care is an important focus of all dialysis organizations.

"We at *Fresenius Medical Care* remain dedicated to improving the quality of life for dialysis patients…"[9].

"Delivering the best patient care possible is the central objective of ours at *Gambro Healthcare*… Knowledge is power. By providing access to information and giving physicians the tools they need to provide optimal patient care, we're working together to improve the quality of life for the people we serve"[10].

"*Renal Care Group* is dedicated to IMPROVING the quality of life and to optimally care for those patients with chronic and acute renal disease. We are committed to the philosophy that optimal care is attained throughout the application of the state-of-the-art technology, continual quality improvement, staff education, and patient/family education."[11].

"Our goal is complete patient rehabilitation... *DCI's* (Dialysis Clinic, Inc.) philosophy has always been a commitment to patients... The care of the patient is our reason for existence"[12].

"*IDF* (Independent Dialysis Foundation) offers convenient and personalized care from a staff that puts the welfare of the patients first"[13].

These statements suggest that the goals in quality of care for different types of organizations are quite similar. What then are the reasons for observations showing differences in structure, process and outcomes? Economic pressures are real in a constrained Medicare reimbursement system for all types of facilities. For-profit facilities appear to have implemented processes that result in greater efficiency. Some evidence also suggests that non-profit facilities later adopt the practices associated with efficiency introduced by for-profit facilities [4].

This suggests that observed differences in efficiency and quality that exist today may converge over time through the identification and dissemination of information about best practices. Information that reveals the relationship between practice structure, processes of care and outcomes could help in this regard. Such knowledge might help to narrow the differences between non-profit and for-profit facilities in both efficiency and quality of care (Figure VI).

CONCLUSION

Studies suggest that structure, process, and outcome differences in quality of care between for-profit and non-profit dialysis facilities exist. These have also shown that for-profit facilities appear particularly sensitive to fiscal pressures and have achieved higher efficiency. With better outcomes data guiding practices in the face of real economic pressures, decisions about clinical care and resource allocation may lead to optimal outcomes.

Neil R. Powe, MD, MPH, MBA
Director, Welch Center for Prevention, Epidemiology and Clinical Research
The Johns Hopkins Medical Institutions, Baltimore, Maryland

REFERENCES

1. Griffiths, RI. Powe, NR, Gaskins, DJ et al. The production of dialysis by For-Profit and Not for Profit renal dialysis facilities. Health Services Research. 1994;29:475-487.
2. United States Renal Data System 2001 Annual Data Report
3. Powe, NR. Thamer, M et al, Hwang W, Fink NE, Bass EB, Sadler JH, Levin NW. Cost-quality tradeoffs in dialysis care Am J of Kidney Dis. 2002;39:116-26.
4. Agodoa LYC, Wolfe RA and Port FK. Reuse of dialyzers and clinical outcomes: fact or fiction. Am J Kidney Dis. 1998;32 (6 Suppl 4):S88-92.
5. Powe NR, Griffiths R, Anderson G et al. Medicare payment policy and recombinant erythropoietin prescribing for dialysis patients. Am J Kidney Dis. 1993;22:557-567.
6. Garg P, Frick K, Diener-West M, Powe NR. Effect of For-Profit ownership of dialysis facilities on patient survival and referral for transplantation evaluation. N Engl J Med. 1999;341:1653-60.
7. Irvin, RA. Quality of care differences by ownership in United States renal dialysis facilities. ASAIO J. 2000;46(6):775-8.
8. Port el al (2000 letter) N Engl J Med. 2000;342:1053-1056.
9. Fresenius mission statement Website: http://www.fmcag.com/internet/fmc/fmcag/agintpub.nsf/Content/Our+Mission (accessed on 5/24/02)
10. Gambro. Website: http://www.gambro.com/Page.asp?id=2923 (accessed 5/24/02)
11. Renal Care Group. Website: http:www.renalcaregroup.com/html/about_us.htm (accessed 5/24/02).
12. Dialysis Clinic, Inc. Webpage: http://www.dciinc.org/corporate/philosophy.htm (accessed 5/24/02)
13. Independent Dialysis Foundation. Website: http://www.idfdn.org/about.htm (accessed 5/24.02)

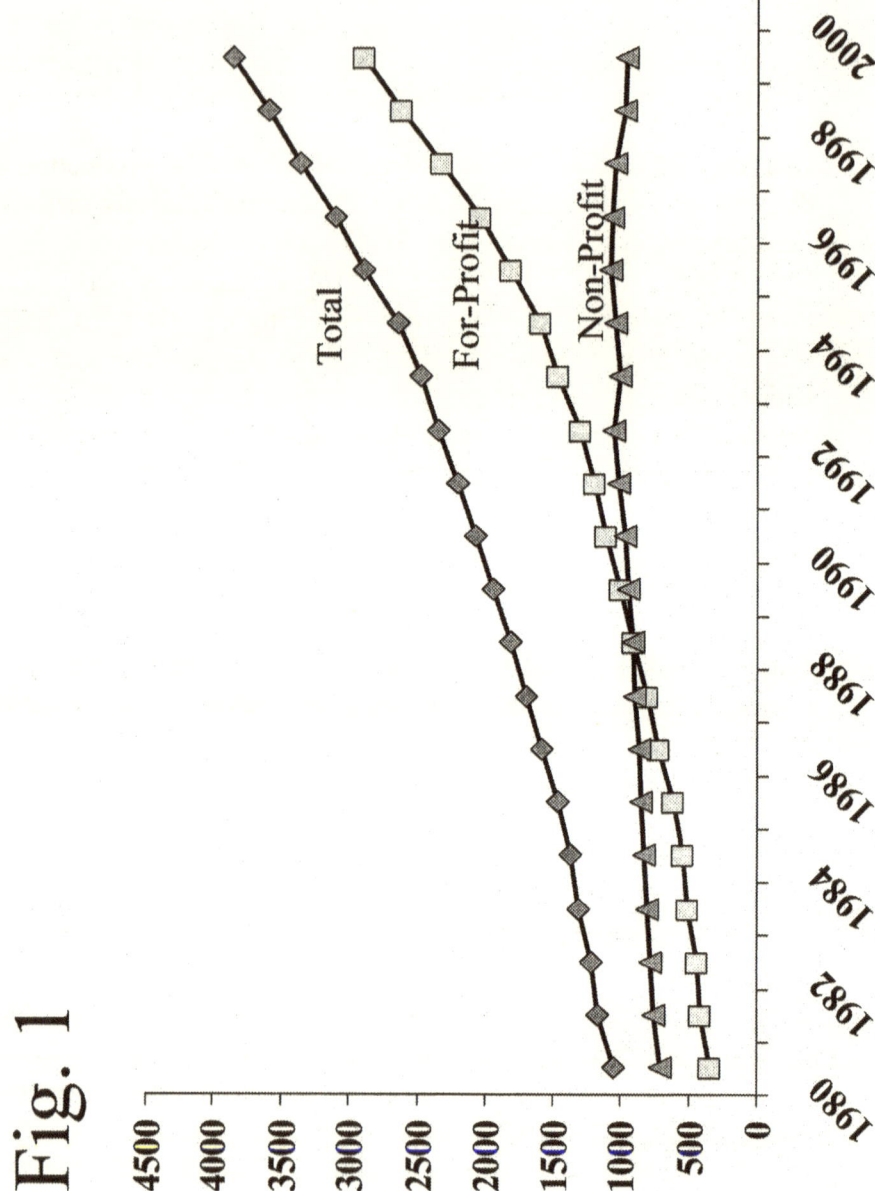

Fig. 1

Fig. 2

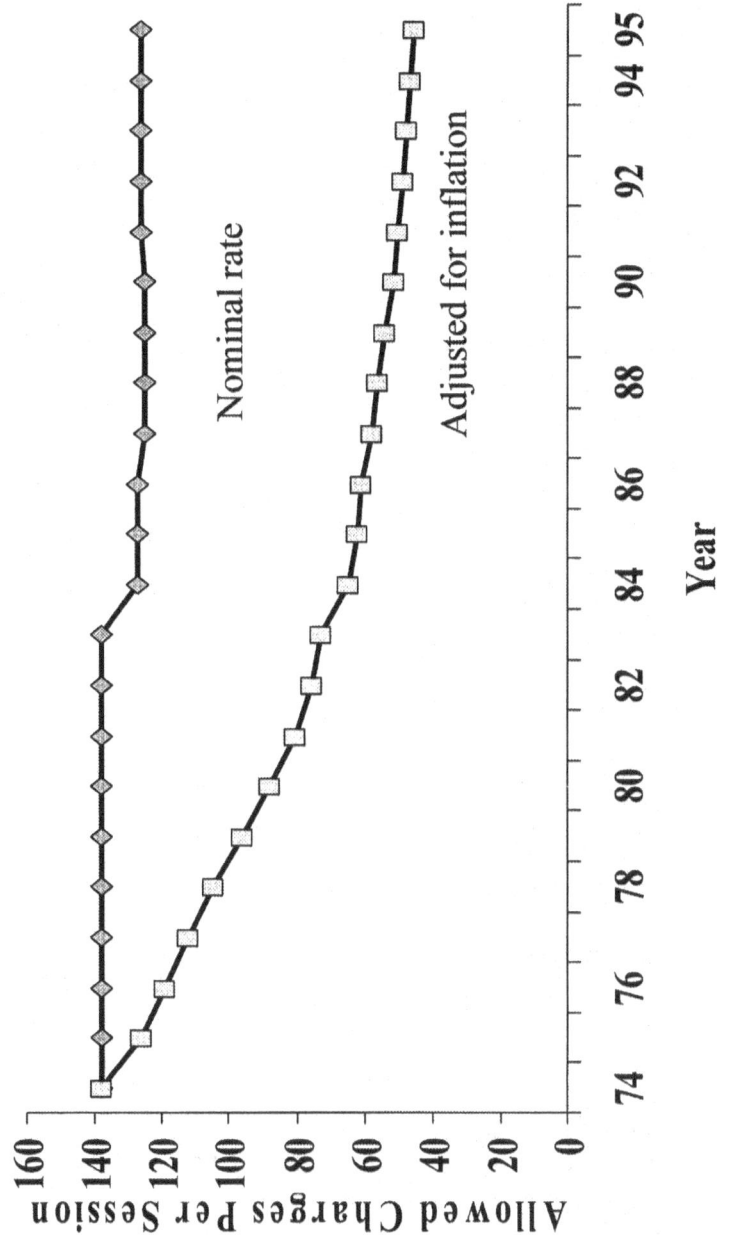

Nominal rate

Adjusted for inflation

Allowed Charges Per Session

Year

Fig. 3

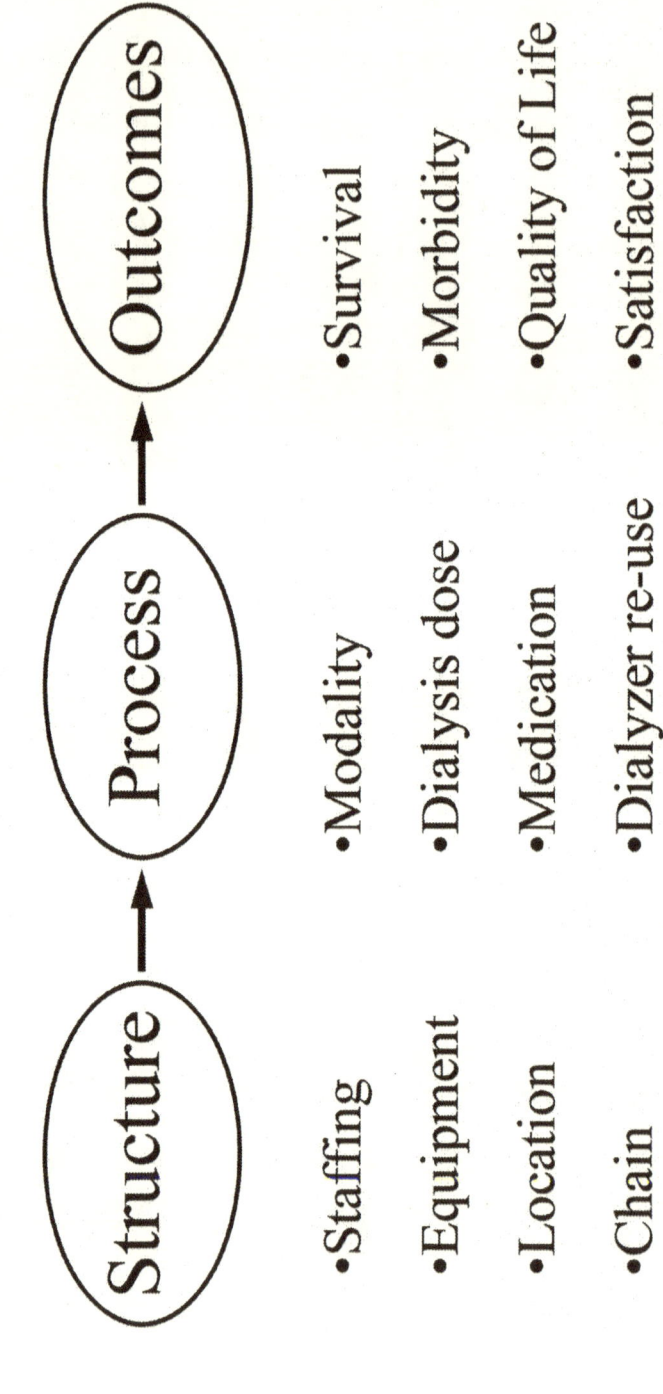

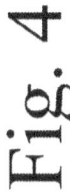

Fig. 4

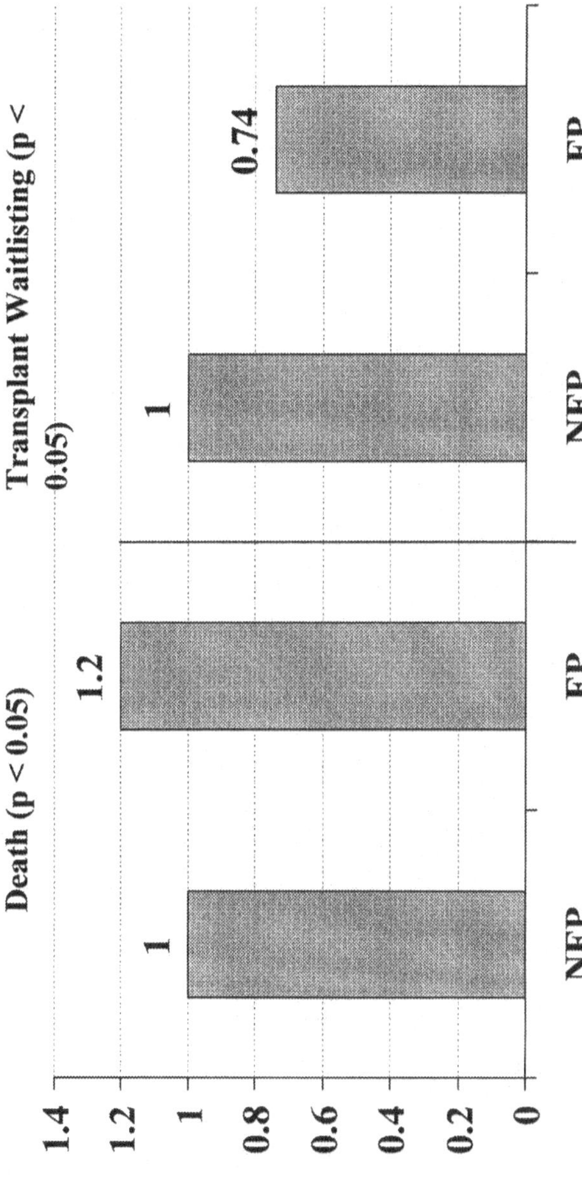

Transplant Waitlisting (p < 0.05)

0.74

FP

1

NFP

Death (p < 0.05)

1.2

FP

1

NFP

1.4
1.2
1
0.8
0.6
0.4
0.2
0

Modified with permission from: Garg P, Frick K, Diener-West M, Powe NR. Effect of For-Profit Ownership of Dialysis Facilities on Patient Survival and Referral for Transplantation Evaluation. *New England Journal of Medicine* 1999; 341: 1653-60

Fig. 5

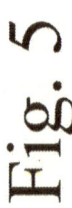

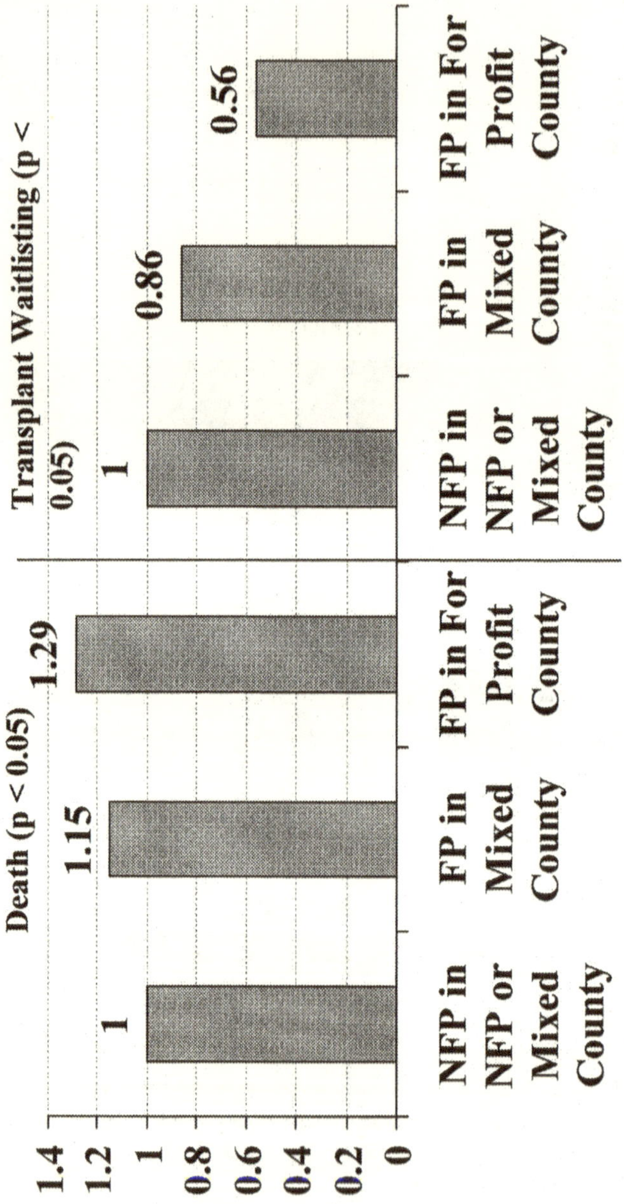

Death (p < 0.05)
Transplant Waitlisting (p < 0.05)
1.4
1.2
1
0.8
0.6
0.4
0.2
0
1
1.15
1.29
1
0.86
0.56
NFP in NFP or Mixed County
FP in Mixed County
FP in For Profit County
NFP in NFP or Mixed County
FP in Mixed County
FP in For Profit County

Modified with permission from: Garg P, Frick K, Diener-West M, Powe NR. Effect of For-Profit Ownership of Dialysis Facilities on Patient Survival and Referral for Transplantation Evaluation. *New England Journal of Medicine* 1999; 341: 1653-60

Fig. 6

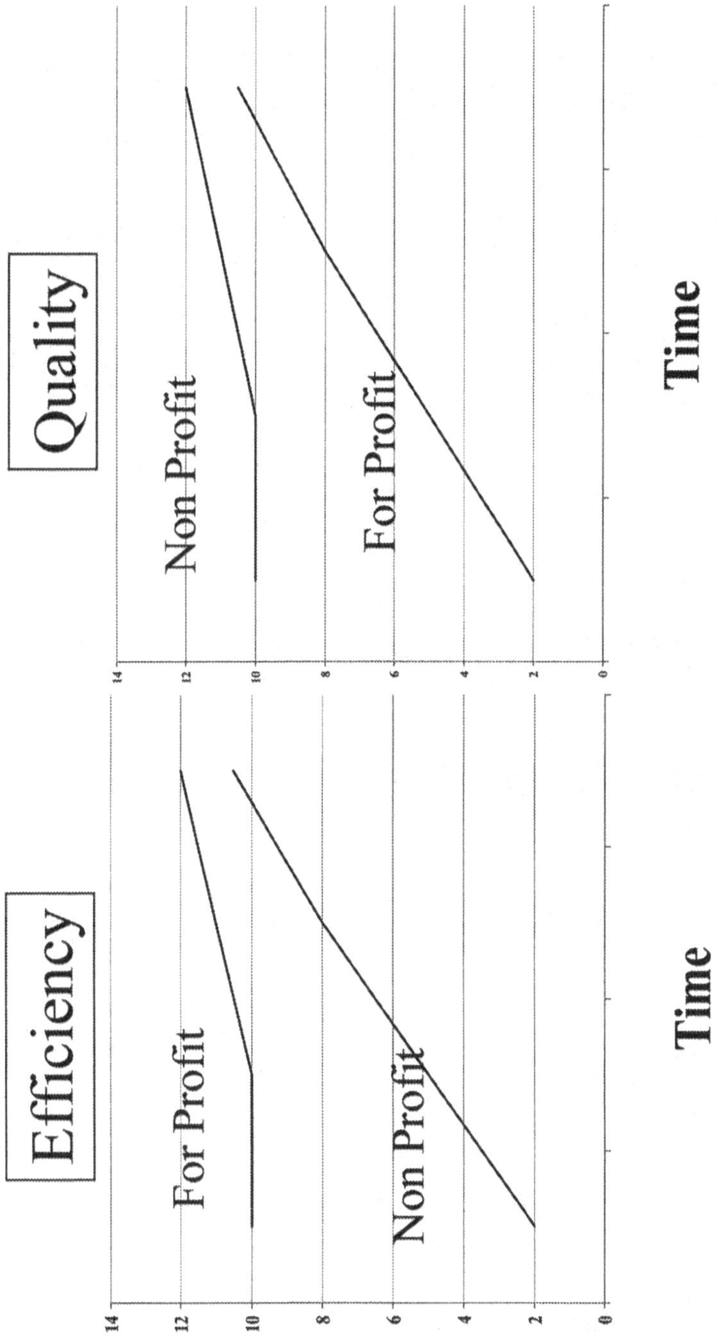

Efficiency

For Profit

Non Profit

Time

Quality

Non Profit

For Profit

Time

Figures Legend:

Fig I: Providers of ESRD in the U.S. (Source: United States Renal Data System)

Fig II: Dialysis Reimbursement Rate – 1974 through 1995 (Source: Center for Medicaid and Medicare Services)

Fig III: Evaluating Quality of Care: Donabedian's Model

Fig IV: Adjusted Relative Hazard of Death and Waitlisting – For Profit vs Not For Profit Facilities (Modified with permission from Garg P, Frick K, Diener-West M, Powe NR. Effect of For-Profit Ownership of Dialysis Facilities on Patient Survival and Referral for Transplantation Evaluation. New England Journal of Medicine 1999; 341: 1653-60)

Fig V: Adjusted Relative Hazard of Death and Waitlisting by Profit Status and Composition of All Facilities in County (Modified with permission from Garg P, Frick K, Diener-West M, Powe NR. Effect of For-Profit Ownership of Dialysis Facilities on Patient Survival and Referral for Transplantation Evaluation. New England Journal of Medicine 1999; 341: 1653-60)

Fig VI: Hypothetical Scenarios for Efficiency and Quality of Dialysis Providers

Is Dietary Counseling Effective in a Multicultural Setting?

Joan D. Mayers, MS, RN, CNN

Introduction

Nutritional counseling is vital towards the success of the hemodialysis prescription. Presented here are exerps from a study that illustrates this point. The study design is qualitative. It investigates and describes the lived experiences of dietary restrictions in English-speaking, West Indian (WI) adults on maintenance hemodialysis. A phenomenological approach was used to interview the five sample patients from the Chronic Hemodialysis Unit at an inner-city hospital. Each subject had a tape-recorded interview with the researcher. Qualitative methods were used to analyze and interpret all data from which the following themes emerged: (a) diet is a major problem; (b) patients adapt by trial and error; (c) WI foods are not listed in the renal failure diets; (d) patients believe that staff lack sufficient knowledge about WI diet and foods; (e) patients believe that eating an American renal diet made them feel worse; and (f) both staff and patients need information on WI foods. The current food list available to the WI hemodialysis patient is insufficient. There is a knowledge deficit regarding WI dietary patterns and their modification for patients on hemodialysis. Further collaborative research is clearly indicated. The findings from this study will add knowledge and understanding in caring for the renal failure population as their numbers steadily increase within multicultural groups.

Nutritional counseling is a significant component in the self-management of patients receiving maintenance hemodialysis therapy. Lee et al. [1] documented that although there appears to be a consensus in the counseling literature that the traditional counselor role fails to meet the needs of consumers in a multicultural setting, there is a mere handful of references that provided counselors with the necessary skills to foster integration of multicultural issues in the counseling industry. For the purposes of this paper, culture is defined as the total of human behavior communicated from generation to generation. Groiler Webster International Dictionary and Feinstein [2,3] state that the choice of categories and amounts of foods pose a large challenge. Patieints are constantly reminded of the seriousness of their illness when faced with dietary restrictions. Beutler et al. [4], state that patients on chronic hemodialysis are continually challenged by their ability to maintain adequate nutrition status. Dietary restrictions take on further significance when clients are given dietary plans that do not reflect their cultural needs and practices.

The Department of City Planning Report (Department of City Planning, 1996) [5], revealed that West Indian (WI) immigrants are highly represented in New York City (NYC) and that this group is a major force in driving the economic engine of growth in New York. Two-thirds of the 562,988 legal immigrants who arrived in NYC from 1992 to 1994 settled primarily in Brooklyn, an inner-city. Gopaul-McNicol [6] stated that 58.5% of WI lived in Brooklyn. Kings County and State University Hospital are the main medical resources in the area, which provide the medical care for the majority of this population. This growing English-speaking WI population comprises a significant percentage of hemodialysis patients, a fact verified by Kinds County Hospital Center (KCHC) dialysis data bank which reported that approximately 34% of the maintenance hemodialysis patients are WI adults (N. John, personal communication, February 10, 1997), while a 44.4% population was reported at State Universitiy Hospital (SUH) (J. Party, personal communication, February 15, 1997).

Little is known about these patients who are on maintenance hemodialysis and their views/perceptions of dietary restrictions. While there are many studies that addressed dietary restrictions in hemodialysis patients [1-12], only one was specific to WI adults [13], and none described the lived experiences. Identification of lived experiences would help caregivers to understand the success and challenges of this heterogeneous group as it relates to living with hemodialysis. The approach may minimize or alleviate patient concerns related to dietary stressors that are associated with this chronoic illness.

Information extrapolated from shared experiences may be useful in generating new knowledge and insight for nephrology nurses who function primarily as clinicians, patient advocates, educators, and as change agents in the patient care focus team. The nurse is in a key position to assess knowledge deficits and to be innovative when developing and implementing creative teaching strategies related to diet. Nurses are challenged to teach and to reinforce dietary restrictions in WI patients who frequently eat ethnic dishes that are quite different from classic American cuisine. Hence, the goal of this study is to gain understanding from the WI perspective of what it is like to be on maintenance hemodialysis with the daily constraints of adhering to the medically prescribed dietary regimen. In addition, this study aims to provide a description of the lived experience of the meaning of dietary restrictions of English-speaking WI adults on maintenance hemodialysis.

Conceptual Framework

This study was guided by Parse's Theory of Human Becoming [14]. The theory focuses on the process of human-health interrelationships. This is the only nursing theory that views paradoxical processes as part of human nature. These paradoxes are viewed as a natural rhythmic occurrence in life. The principles derived from Parse's assumption state that humans produce what is real for them based on choices that they make. As various experiences evolve, people live these beliefs as they interpret them. Humans live in rhythm with the universe. They co-constitute patterns of how they relate to various experiences through paradoxical activities. Parse [14] also made reference to freedom and limitation.

According to her theory, people place value on certain life events and cherish those beliefs/concepts. Individuals should not be told what choices to make; rather there should be a quest to determine the individual's vision, which will lead to a clearer understanding of one's expectations. With this in mind, caregivers may be better equipped to assist the patient in modifying their diet with food preferences and practice. For example, WIs prepared daily cultural staple foods like yams, breadfruit, sweet potatoes, dasheen, edoes and cassava, to name a few of the ground provisions (tuberous roots) whose chemical compositions are still not fully known. They also enjoy many fruits like mangoes, sapodilla, plums, downs, cymite pomcyrye, and vegetables like callaloo. Potassiuma nd phosphorous are other areas of concern to the WI diet because their content still needs to be studied and documented.

Review of the Literature

Current literature focuses on the experiences of researchers with varied degrees of low protein dietary intake, catabolism, protein calorie malnutrition, and strategies for improving dietary compliance in end stage renal disease (ESRD) patients [7-12]. The findings reported were mainly from quantitative studies based on anthropometrics measurements and biochemical parameters.

Berg et al. [15], and Lassiter [16] examined renal diets for American Blacks. The general conclusion of these researchers' findings is that frequently these diets were not tailored to specifically address the cultural practices of the diverse Black population. Wilkie et al.[13], provided the only study that reported on a renal diet for Caribbean patients on maintenance hemodialysis. The researchers reported that industrially prepared renal foods, though available, were too expensive for natives of Jamaica. These foods were tested for palatability and they found taste to be acceptable. Subsequently, the researchers developed a Caribbean renal diet and recipes consisting of local staple crops (dasheen, cassava, arrowroot).

Their aim was to show that locally grown foods could be used to formulate a diet suitable for patients with renal failure. Ironicallly, there was no mention of the use of this diet in patients with renal failure or patients on maintenance hemodialysis. The problem concerning WI patients on hemodialysis was aptly stated by Garraway [17] as she commented, "If you are an ERSD patient of Caribbean origin, you are constantly challenged with the problem of complying with the renal diet while still enjoying your traditional foods".

In WI communities, food products were influenced by the British colonizers, African slaves, East Indian indentured laborers, and the British who prefer hot foods made extra spicy with curry, nutmeg, ginger, and coconut milk. Other coconut products are also a regular staple of WI cooking. Pigeon peas and rice are to the WI what meat and potatoes are to Americans. The combination of coconut milk and hot pepper with meals provides both richness and bite. In the WI culture, Sunday lunch is very special and lavish. WI eat large amounts of meat, fish, and highly seasoned foods that have high sodium content. This group also consumes a variety of fruits, which are possibly high sources of potassium.

Design and Methodology

Parse's qualitative phenomenological design was chosen because its main purpose is to describe the lived experience of people regarding a phenomenon [14]. Excerpts from the actual interviews were used to validate the essence of the experience that the participant described.

Sample

This study consisted of five participants (three man and two women) who receive maintenance hemodialysis therapy. Each was born on an English-speaking WI island and their age ranged between 22 and 50 years. At the time of the interview none of the subjects were hospitalized.

A purposive nonprobability sampling technique was used to select the study population. Participants were interviewed until no new themes or patterns emerged. The study was then closed.

Data collection

Following IRB approval, the researcher contacted eligible patients. Participants who agreed to be part of the study signed an informed consent. The purpose of the study was then explained and confidentiality of the data insured. An audiotaped interview was conducted in a private placae at a convenient time for the participants. Semistructured interviewed techniques were used and each participant completed a short demographic questionnaire consisting of four items. The main interview question asked was, would you explain to me how you live with the dietary restrictions of hemodialysis on a daily basis? When indicated, probing questions/phrases were used for the purpose of clarification.

Data analysis.

All data was analyzed using a constant comparative method. Each transcript was read and a chronological number was assigned to each new pattern. Each statement was assigned a number that corresponded. The patient's views were sought to establish internal validity. The researcher reviewed the transcribed interview with the subjects to determine whether they felt the essential message was clearly communicated or understood by the researcher.

Results

When the quotes were analyzed for emerging key and recurrent ideas or
events, six themes emerged from the data. The themes were as
follows:

2. **Diet was a major problem**

Mr. T&T exclaimed, *Naturally it is a very depressing time. It does affect
you. You know longer have the freedom to eat anything that you feel to eat.
The liquids, that is a hard one. Oh, Gosh.*

Mr. SVG responded by listing the foods he likes to eat, *...breadfruit,
callaloo, and sometimes yam, dasheen plantain, bananas, and
things like that. I feel restricted because most of these things I would
like to eat on a daily basis. I don't know, it's like I am missing a lot of
things that I could have been eating if I did not have kidney disease
problems.*

Patients experienced depression and difficulties in food selection. Mr.
SVG likewise felt that he was missing out on many of his favorite foods.

3. **Patients adapted by trial and error**

According to Ms. T&T, *Some things I follow and some things I eat and I
don't really know the contents of them. Like ground provision you will know
what is high or low in potassium because we eat a lot of ground provision,
right, like dasheen and yam. Well, I know about the plantain because I eat
a piece sometimes. I eat the WI food but I really don' know much about
what's on the diet.*

Mr. T&T stated, *In the beginning, it was difficult. Naturally, because
of you know living in a house with a lot of people. If I have to eat certain
things, naturally my kids might not want to eat that, so my wife used to end
up cooking different foods.* These problems seemed to be linked to trial and
error efforts to adjust the diet to family practices. At first, the regimen was
very strict, but over time they were able to add certain foods if eaten in small
portions. They learned to adjust to the requirements of social living where
everyone had their own tastes and desires. Likewise, Ms. T & T indicated
that she made judgements as to its potassium content. She suspected that
ground products had higher potassium content than did greens.

4. **WI foods were not listed in the diet.**

Mr. SVG said, *I know that dietitians try their best. I guess a list is given
because if you tell someone to have a little bit of this, they think that they
can go home and have a lot.* Ms. T&T said she *drinks grapefruit juice*

sometimes, especially the one that is canned in Trinidad. There are many WIs who come to the clinic but the food list is more American.

Standard diet therapy for hemodialysis was unrelated to the WI culture and lifestyles. These patients felt that a list was given to be used as a guide for better diet control but it failed to serve its purpose because the typical foods of the WI people were not incorporated into the list that was distributed to them. They were also of the opinion that the food represented a typical American food list.

5. **Patients believed that staff did not know about WI food and diets.**

According to Mr. Barbados, *Well, you know because it is not listed anywhere and, in some cases, the names are different. For instance, if something in the United States is called by a different name from the name that I know it by, although it is something that I know, I don't know if it is something that I can eat because of the difference in the name, then I would either think I could have it or that I can't have it.*

All participants were concerned about the fact that the staff did not seem to know what foods in the participants' WI diet should be regulated and that the cultural names of the foods should be listed (e.g., yucca is the same item as cassava). In different islands, one food item has various names.

6. **Patients believed that eating American renal diet made them feel worse.**

Mr. Barbados stated, *Well, I started following it and then I found out that I used to be weaker and stuff like tehat, so that's when I started eating my regular foods.* Ms. Jamaica added, *Well the food they tell you to eat, it have no substance. It make you feel so weaky, weaky. If you could eat some of your back home food, maybe you could have a little strength in your body. But these food they have no taste. And especially being a diabetic, you have to give up everything. They say don't eat potatoes or soup because the potatoes have potassium and the soup have too much liquid and I like soup.*

Ms. J felt that the food that was allowed on the diet did not seem to provide her with enough energy. By regular foods Mr. Barbados alluded to cultural foods like, *yams, sweet potatoes, dasheen, breadfruit, pumpkin, and stuff like that.* The key to the subjective definition of WI food was referred to here as regular food and North American food as that which made them feel weak or weaky weakyk according to Ms. Jamaica.

7. **There is a great need for information on native foods.**

Mr. SVG believes, *"I think this will be helpful to the new patients starting on dialysis if something could be done to help put some back home foods on the list and let the dietitians learn about our foods, like which is high in potassium and so on. And then maybe you can tell us abouat it when we are on the machine."* Ms. Jamaica reported, *I guess white people made it and the patients they are white too. Another thing is that they probably don't know about our type of food and cooking because most time those people go on vacation in the Caribbean and they don't really know how things are prepared, they eat it and it tastes good. It would be good if they could include some of our foods on the list that they give when you go on dialysis.*

In this theme we see that, on the one hand, patients are dependent on the dietitian to provide them with information relative to the maintenance of appropriate eating habits and, on the other hand, realize that the dietitians they depend upon do not know about their native diet. And as Ms. Jamaica said, *the teaching material was made by white dietitians for white patients.* Because there is a definite shift in the current patient population, there is a need to change the teaching contents to accommodate their needs. It would seem that (a) it would be easy to develop a list of WI foods and the mineral contents of each by an informed dietician, (b) apparently one exists, and (c) such a list has not been adequately distributed to WI dialysis patients. The findings suggest that dialysis patients have difficulty maintaining the strict demands of diets necessary for successful dialysis. WI patients have additional problems because they wish to maintain their traditional diets and eating habits. One problem is that the WI diet has high levels of potassium, which is restricted in dialysis. The response of the health care system to the problem of WI patients has not been systematic and has occurred primarily on an ad hoc basis.

Discussion

The research literature indicated that diets of non-European ethnic groups are understudied [13,15-17]. The findings of this study are in agreement with this conclusion. Four of the five respondents in this study had to engage in trial-and-error techniques to integrate their native eating habits with the demands of hemodialysis. Only one respondent was provided a list of WI foods and their contents. This lack of proper information can be considered poor health care practice, especially as diet maintenance can be life threatening among hemodialysis patients.

The respondents voiced a considerable amount of frustration when recounting their feelings towards integration of native foods to maintain adequate labs for hemodialysis.

One very important aspect of the problem was the unavailability of information concerning the criteria a WI hemodialysis patient must consider when making food selections. For example, a publication from the National Kidney Foundation [18] specified the criteria for American, Mexican, Italian, and Asian ethnic foods, but for the hemodialysis patient there was no mention of WI foods.

Implications

Nursing Practice

The results of the study suggest that having a list of WI foods and their chemical composition is critical to the care of WI hemodialysis patients. Nephrology nurses play a vital role in the lives of the patients and their families. More information will enhance education. Whenever hemodialysis patients are identified as WIs, they should receive a list of WI foods and their contents. The data suggests that a piecemeal approach is ineffective. There should be a policy indicating that all patients from all ethnic groups receive lists of their native foods complete with contents. This approach would help patients and their families develop the skills that are necessary to maintain proper self-care.

When properly implemented, the new information will help to increase adherence to the prescribed dietary regimen. This will heighten the awareness that there is a need to find out more information about as many diets as possible and to better understand how patients from various cultures cope with their prescribed renal diet. It was indicated here that a conversion list would be very useful in affording more appropriate food selections. This should provide improved understanding of the dietary education function of nursing and may help to improve patient compliance. The availability of a multicultural food list would facilitate patients in functioning at their highest possible level in rehabilitation and related nutrition efforts.

Nursing Education

The most important implication of the findings involves educating nurses and dietitians about the dietary needs of WI patients and the need to convert WI foods to meaningful portion control to enable hemodialysis patients to follow a healthy diet. These efforts would entail the development and implementation of dietary awareness programs for nurses specifically geared towards WI patients who are on hemodialysis. The nephrology nurse specialist can increase personal knowledge of WI foods so that patients can be educated concerning the chemical composition, portion control, and proper frequency of intake of these foods needed to remain healthy. Once successful, this strategy could be employed using a multicultural group.

Nursing Research

Education designed for determining how to property advise WI patients on their renal diet may make a tremendous impact on patient care by yielding positive outcomes and fostering a higher degree of patient satisfaction. Since the number of WI adults receiving maintenance hemodialysis is increasing, there is a need to raise the consciousness of the nephrology nurses regarding cultural influences associated with diet and health affecting nursing education and practice. Such a program should be evaluated in terms of its effect on the attitudes toward disseminating ethnic-based dietary information and knowledge of the composition of ethnic foods gained by nurses in the program.

The small sample of this study does not allow generalization of the results to the hemodialysis community at large. Further research is necessary, employing larger sample sizes and greater controls to study ethnic dietary practices of hemodialysis patients from non—European backgrounds. Development of continuous education programs for staff and more structured patient education programs, patient education groups, and application of research grants towards this topic should be instituted and evaluated.

Counseling

Some patients may feel more comfortable with staff members who share the same cultural background as themselves. If the counselor is from a different background as the patient they should be honest and make referrals soothe patient could get the appropriate help and information. Another approach is for both patients and staff to share information from their communities so both groups can become more aware of the practices of the two groups. The development and implementation of multicultural nutritional awareness programs will also assist this process. Both groups may consider identifying new opportunities to learn about each other's culture. One more alternate is for the patient as well the patients from the various cultural background to use themselves a model to address the concept of multiculturalism within the group.

Conclusion

The findings also indicate that the distribution of lists of foods available to the WI hemodialysis patient and nursing efforts at education regarding the impact of eating their ethnic foods is not sufficient to provide an adequate level of health. Thus, many WI patients are unaware of the dangers of certain foods, certain portion sizes, and frequency of intake in lieu of keeping with their ethnic customs concerning these foods until it interferes with their dialysis. This is not necessarily a purposeful action of WI patients, since the findings indicate the information is not made available. Since the number of hemodialysis patients is increasing and a large percentage of these patients are from the West Indies, the findings show that this should be considered a topic of critical concern.

Additionally, the findings indicate that WI hemodialysis patients are frustrated with the problems of maintaining appropriate diets for hemodialysis with lack of adequate information about thei rnative foods. The data suggest that, in some cases, patients monitor their own physiological responses to various foods in lieu of scienteific information. Respondents indicated the wish to have a listing of WI foods that shows their composition so they could have a guide to help them maintain proper diets. Because the use of good is a manner of promoting the acculturation process, it is a natural form of manifestation in various multicultural groups. According to Alexander et al. [19], "Counselors have been struggling to delineate the "how to" of multicultural counseling, and although some direction has been provided in the literature, much is left unsaid or left up to the imagination. What we have attempted to illustrate is that counselors can tap into the minority client's everyday life to aid in the therapeutic process....".

Recommendations

The results of this study show a need for a study that investigates the sentiments of hemodialysis patients towards their dietary restriction. Research needs to be conducted by nephrology nurses in U. S. hospitals that serve WI patients on their knowledge of the composition of WI foods and their teaching skills of imparting dietary knowledge of their WI patients. In addition, studies need to be conducted in collaboration with nurses and dietitians on dietary issues for non-European ethnic patients.

The preliminary study conducted by this researcher should provide a foundation for future studies related to experience of the WI and their hemodialysis diet regimen. This study can be replicated using any cultural group whose foods need further exploration. The following topics were extracted from the list of research recommendations published by the National Kidney Foundation DOQI (2000). A better understanding of the effects of nutrition intervention counseling methods on various aspects of nutrition; The indications for nutritional support in the dialysis patient; Evaluate the effects of Intraperitoneal feeding on physical function; Evaluate strategies to enhance compliance with particular emphasis on the adolescent age group; Would adaptation of a nutritional tool specifically for the pediatric population be useful for evaluating nutrition status of children.

One can safely infer that further interdisciplinary research is clearly indicated. It is imperative to utilize a qualitative design for better appreciation of the nutritional way of life of the various cultural/ethnic groups of patient that we serve. After some of the recommended research have been completed and documented, our patients could experience a more effective nutritional counseling since more pertinent information and skills will be more available to the healthcare providers. This newly acquired information will be evident as the patients incorporate more and more of their cultural food into their daily diets with added confidence. Then and only then can we stand a chance to operationalize the Multicultural Counseling Competencies by the Association for Multicultural Counseling and Development and use them as a benchmark for effective multicultural nutrition counseling.

References

1. Lee CC, Richardson BL(Eds). Multicultural issies in counseling: New approaches to diversity. 1991. Alexandria., VA: American Counseling Association.

2. The New Groiler Webster International Dictionary of the English Language.

3. Feinstein EI. Nutritional therapy in maintenance hemodialysis. Nutritional Management, 1993;17:197-198. http://cc.byc.edu/ causes/sw660/readings/Creative Approaches.htm pg 1-8

4. Beutler KT, Park GK, Wilkowski M J. Effect of oral supplementation on nutrition indicators in hemodialysis patients. Journal of Renal Nutrition 1997;7(2):77-82.

5. Department of City Planning. 1996. The newest New Yorkers. New York: Author.

6. Gopaul-McNicol S. Working with West Indian Families. New York: Guilford Press, 1993.

7. Chang C Y, Green GW. Dialysis compliance among hemodialysis patients. Diabetes and Transplantation 1994;11:184-189.

8. Colombi A, Martin R. Nutrition in kidney disease. Schweizerishe Rundschau fur Medizin Praxis 1991;80(40):1062-1065.

9. DeMotte C. Renal nutrition and the noncompliant patient: Some guidelines. Nephrology News & Issues, 1990;4(11):14,16,54.

10. Devine W. Review of nutritional status and diet in dialysis and renal transplant patients. Dialysis and Transplantation 1994;1:38-46.

11. Hood SS, Loney N. Anthropometrics for dialysis patients. Renal Nutrition Forum, Spring, 1994.

12. Mitch W E. Dietary protein restriction in chronic renal failure: Nutrition efficacy, compliance, and progression of renal insufficiency. J Am Soc Nephrol 1991;2(4), 823-831.

13. Wilkie H, Landman J, Jackson A, Chir B, Picou D. A Caribbean diet for the management of renal failure. West Indian Medical Journal 1982;31(1):20-28.

14. Parse RR. Illuminations: The Human Becoming Theory in Practice

and Research. New York: National League for Nursing, 1995.

15. Berg J, Berg B L. Compliance, diet, and cultural factors among black Americans with end-stage renal disease. journal of National Black Nurses Association 1989;3(2):16-28.

16. Lassiter SM. Black is a color, not a culture: Implications for health care. ABNF Journal, 1994;5(1):4-9.

17. Garraway E. Caribbean food. Renalife 1990;5(2):14-15.

18. National Kidney Foundation. Dining Out With Confidence: A Guide for Renal Patients. (Pamphlet) 1995, New York.

19. Alexander C, Sussman L. Creative Approaches of Multicultural Counseling K T, Park G K, Wilkowski M J. Effect or oral supplementation on nutrition indicators in hemodialysis patients. Journal of Renal Nutrition 1997;7(1):77-82.

Joan D. Mayers
Quality Management
Department of Nursing
SUNY Downstate Medical Center
Brooklyn, New York

Racial Differences in Transplant Outcomes: Biology vs. Socioeconomic Factors

Moro O. Salifu, MD, FACP

Introduction

Renal transplantation affords a better quality of life than dialysis therapy, however there are differences in outcomes between Whites and non-whites. The differences appear to stem from a complex interplay in both biologic and socioeconomic factors. Though this chapter will attempt to outline some of the published data on this subject, it should be noted that knowledge of how these factors interplay is still not fully understood.

It should also be noted that the available data does not contain information on all racial groups, limiting most of the assessment to Blacks and Whites. The chapter begins with establishing that there are racial differences in access to renal transplantation, acute rejections, graft and patient survival and comorbidity such as posttransplant diabetes. Following this would be a discussion of potential biologic and socioeconomic reasons for the differences.

Differences in access to renal transplantation

Renal transplantation is a process involving a series of steps related to medical suitability interest in transplantation, pre-transplantation workup and moving up the waiting list to eventual transplantation [1]. Blacks and other racial groups are less likely to be wait-listed for cadaveric renal transplantation than Whites [1-3]. Although Blacks and Whites are equally medically suitable, Blacks are less likely to proceed throughout the steps as compared with Whites.

Data from the United Network for Organ Sharing (UNOS) show

significant racial differences in all the measures of access to renal transplantation [3]. For instance, the 1999 annual data of the UNOS database indicate that Whites had higher rates of wait listing, living/cadaver donations, and living/cadaver recipients than Blacks, Hispanics and Asians. Whites also have lower rates of HLA mismatched kidneys [4] as compared with Blacks (1.8±6 vs 3±1, p<0.001).

Differences in clinical outcomes

The risk of graft loss due to chronic allograft failure, acute rejection and graft loss due to all causes in Blacks in 1.8, 1.3 and 1.2 respectively, with a surprisingly lower rate of death due to infections in Blacks as compared with Whites [5]. In the study reported by Butkus et al. [4], Blacks were twice as likely to experience an acute rejection as compared with Whites (34.8% vs 19.4%, p<0.05) over a two-year period. Data from the United States Renal data System [6] show that, the 12-year graft survival in Blacks in significantly lower than Whites or other races combined. Posttransplant diabetes, a common complication of steroid and calcineurin inhibitor therapy, and hypertension occur more frequently in Blacks than in whites [7,8].

Reasons for these differences

There is no single satisfactory explanation for these differences in transplant outcomes. Both socioeconomic and biologic factors are intricately involved. The differences do not appear to arise from differences in type of immunosuppression, type of transplant or referral by nephrologist. Neylan et a, [7] showed that patient and graft survival of cyclosporine or tacrolimus treated patients were similar. Similarly, Meier-Kriesche et al, showed that Blacks did equally well on cellcept [9] and the interleukin 2 receptor blocker daclizumab [10].

Ojo et al. [11], showed that both Black and White renal transplant recipients showed a greater than 50% reduction in the risk of allograft loss at all points up to 5 years posttransplant, w hen living donor kidneys were chosen over cadaveric kidney transplantation, though the cumulative risk of graft failure is higher in Blacks than all other races [6,12]. Referral for transplantation by Nephrologists does not also appear to account for the difference in outcome between Blacks and Whites, though Asian men are less referred than White men [2,13].

Socioeconomic factors

Socioeconomic factors play a significant role in explaining the differences in access to renal transplantationa nd clinical outcomes. Kasiske et al. [14], showed that racial and ethnic minorities, those less well educated and those with fewer financial resources were less likely than their counterparts to be placed on the kidney transplant wwaiting list befor einitiation of dialysis.

At the time transplantation, Butkus et al. [3], reported lower mean annual income in Blacks compared with whites (US$ 10396.00 vs. US$ 18127.00, p<0.05), higher number of patients below the federal poverty level in Blacks compared with Whites (58% vs. 31%, p<0.05), lower number of y ears of education in Blacks compared with whites (11.2+2.5 vs. 12.4+3, p<0.05), lower rate of private insurance plus Medicare (15.7 vs. 43.6%, p<0.05) but higher number of Medicaid plus Medicare (65.1 vs. 33.0%, p<0.05). Noncompliance was more prevalent in Blacks than in Whites. In this study, the 4-year graft survival of Blacks above the federal poverty level was equivalent to Whites below or above the federal poverty level (91 vs 90% or 89%) with Blacks below the federal poverty level having the worse graft survival (68%). Regardless of race, poverty per se, results in reduced renal allograft survival [15], thus it seems that the real issue is financial resources, which is poor in minority recipients as shown above.

Biologic factors

The immune system has generally been considered stronger in Blacks than Whites. Several reasons provide for this consideration. Blacks have higher rates of acute rejection, chronic allograft rejection and overall shorter kidney graft survival than Whites [4-6]. Furthermore, it has been shown that mixed lymphocyte response is higher in Blacks htan whites [16], suggesting a heightened immune response. It has also been shown that steroid clearance is actually decreased in Blacks [17] and they also require higher doses of tacrolimus [18] in order to achieve blood levels as in non-Blacks. It is certain that Blacks metabolize tacrolimus differently though the mechanism is unknown at this time. These latter biologic differences may account for the higher incidence of toxic side effects of steroid and calcineurin inhibitors such as diabetes hypertension, hyperlipidemia and cardiovascular disease.

The higher rates of acute and chronic rejection as well as overall lower graft survival may not be attributable to a stronger immune system alone, but rather a combination of a strong immune system which is inadequately suppressed. Data from Meier-Kriesche et al show that Blacks die less from infectious causes than Whites [5] but have worse graft survival than whites [6], suggesting inadequate immunosuppression in Blacks. Blacks may require more immunosuppression than Whites to achieve equivalent long-term graft survival, however, this is limited because of the higher rates of toxic side effects. A future approach, tailoring immunosuppression by race appears prudent.

Another biologic factor with a strong link to graft survival is hypertension. 48.3% of Black renal transplant recipients have hypertension as a primary cause of ESRD whereas only 6.1% of Whites have hypertension as the primary diagnosis [8]. The 6-year graft survival of a Black normotensive (MAP =107 mmHg) is equivalent to Whites with or without hypertension whereas the Black hypertensives have the worse survival. Though Blacks have higher incidence of posttransplant diabetes and hypercholesterolemia, there is no evidence that they impact on graft survival.

Taken together, the evidence presented above suggests a complex relationship between socioeconomic and biologic factors in renal transplant outcomes. Blacks are more likely than other racial groups in these studies to have low income, education, insurance, employment but a higher incidence of hypertension and evidence suggesting a heightened immune system, which is under suppressed. All these impact on the outcomes discussed above.

Moro O. Salifu, MD, FACP
Renal Disease Division
Department of Medicine
SUNY Downstate Medical Center
Brooklyn, New York

References

1. Alexander GC, Sehgal AR. Barriers to cadaveric renal transplantation among Blacks, women and the poor. JAMA 1998;280:1148-1152.
2. Wolfe RA, Ashby VB, Milford EL, Bloembergen WE, Agodoa LY, Held PJ. Port FK. Differences in access to cadaveric renal transplantation in the United States. Am J Kidney Dis 2000;36: 1025-1033.
3. United Network for Organ Sharing (UNOS) Annual Report, 2000, www.unos.org/data/anrpt00
4. Butkus DE, Dottes Al. Meydrech EF, Barber WH. Effect of poverty and other socioeconomic variables on renal allograft survival. Transplantation 2001;72:261-2666.
5. Meier-Kriesche HU, Ojo A. Magee JC, Cibrik DM, Hanson JA, Leichtman AB, Kaplan B. African-American renal transplant recipients experience decreased risk of death due to infection: possible implications for immunosuppressive strategies. Transplantation 2000;70:375-9.
6. US Renal Data System: USRDS 2000 Annual Data Report, The National Institute of Health, National Institute of Diabetes and Digestive and Kidney Diseases, Bethesda, MD, June 2000.
7. Neylan JF. Effect of race and immunosuppression in renal transplantation: three-year survival results from a US multicenter, randomized trial. FK506 Kidney Transplant Study Group. Transplant Proc 1998;30:1355-1358.
8. Cosio RI, Dillon JJ. Falkenhain ME, Tesi RJ, Henry ML, Elkhammas EA, Davies EA, Bumgardner GI, Ferguson RM. Racial differences in renal allograft survival: the role of systemic hypertension. Kidney Int 1995;47:1136-1141.
9. Meier-Kriesche HU, Ojo AO, Leichtman AB, Punch JD, Hanson JA, Cibrik DM, Kaplan B. Effect of mycophenolate mofetil on long-term outcomes in African American renal transplant recipients. J Am Soc Nephrol 2000;11:2366-2370.
10. Meier-Kriesche HU, Palenkar SS, Friedman GS, Mulgaonkar SP, Goldblat MV, Kaplan B. Efficacy of Daclizumab in an African-

American and Hispanic renal transplant population. Transpl Int 2000;13:142-145.

11. Ojo AO, Port FK, Mauger EA, Wolfe RA, Leichtman AB. Relative impact of donor type on renal allograft survival in black and white recipients. Am J Kidney Dis 1995;25:623-628.

12. Isaacs RB, Nock SL, Spencer CE, Connors AF Jr, Wang XQ, Sawyer R, Lobo PI. Racial disparities in renal transplant outcomes. Am J Kidney Dis 1999;34:706-12.

13. Thamer M, Hwang W, Fink NE, Sadler JH, Bass EB, Levey AS, Brookmeyer R, Powe NR. CHOICE Study. Choices for Healthy Outcomes in Caring for ESRD. U.S. nephrologists' attitudes towards renal transplantation: results from a national survey. Transplantation 2001;71:281-282.

14. Kasiske kBl, London W, Ellison MD. Race and socioeconomic factors influencing early placement on the kidney transplant waiting list. J Am Soc Nephrol 1998;9:2142-7.

15. Kalil RS, Heim-Duthoy KL, Kasiske BL. Patients with a low income have reduced renal allograft survival. Am J Kidney Dis 1992;20:63-69.

16. Hutchings A, Purcell VIM, Benfield MR. Increased costimulatory responses in African- American kidney allograft recipients. Transplantation 2001;71:692-695.

17. Tornatore KKM, Biocevich DM, Reed K, Tousley K, Singh JP, Venuto RC. Methylprednisolone pharmacokinetics, cortisol response, and adverse effects in black and white renal transplant recipients. Transplantation 1995;59:729-736.

18. Fitzsimmons WE, Bekersky I, Dressier D, Raye K, Hodosh F, Mekki Q. Demograhpic considerations in tacrolimus pharmacokinetics. Transplant Proc 1998;30:1359-64.

About the Author

Dr. Onyekachi Ifudu, a board-certified specialist in both internal medicine and nephrology, received his medical degree from the University of Nigeria and completed his Master of Science in Epidemiology at Harvard University. He is an Associate Professor of Medicine and Director of Inpatient Dialysis Services at SUNY Downstate Medical Center, Brooklyn, New York. Over the past 19 years, Dr. Ifudu has worked exclusively in poor and underprivileged neighborhoods (Harlem & Brooklyn, New York) with severe socio-economic and basic health deprivation. He has first-authored over sixty papers in peer-reviewed medical journals, including a State-of-the-Art article in the New England Journal of Medicine on management of patients with end-stage renal disease. His other books include "AIDS and The Kidney", and "Renal Anemia: Conflicts and Controversies".